"Mounting evidence indicates that refined carbohydrates and high glycemic index foods are contributing to the escalating epidemics of obesity and type 2 diabetes worldwide. This dietary pattern also appears to increase the risk of heart disease and stroke. The skyrocketing proportion of calories from added sugars and refined carbohydrates in Westernized diets portends a future acceleration of these trends. *The Glucose Revolution* challenges traditional doctrines about optimal nutrition and the role of carbohydrates in health and disease. Brand-Miller and colleagues are to be congratulated for an eminently lucid and important book that explains the science behind the glycemic index and provides tools and strategies for modifying diet to incorporate this knowledge. I strongly recommend the book to both health professionals and the general public who could use this state-of-the-art information to improve health and well-being."

—JOANN E. MANSON, M.D., DR.P.H., Professor of Medicine, Harvard Medical School, and Co-Director of Women's Health, Division of Preventive Medicine, Brigham and Women's Hospital

■

"Here is at last a book explaining the importance of taking into consideration the glycemic index of foods for overall health, athletic performance, and in reducing the risk of heart disease and diabetes. The book clearly explains that there are different kinds of carbohydrates that work in different ways and why a universal recommendation to 'increase the carbohydrate content of your diet' is plainly simple and scientifically inaccurate. Everyone should put the glycemic index approach into practice."

—ARTEMIS P. SIMOPOULOS, M.D., senior author of *The Omega Diet* and *The Healing Diet* and President, The Center for Genetics, Nutrition and Health, Washington, D.C., on *The Glucose Revolution*

"*The Glucose Revolution* is nutrition science for the 21st century. Clearly written, it gives the scientific rationale for why all carbohydrates are not created equal. It is a practical guide for both professionals and patients. The food suggestions and recipes are exciting and tasty."

—RICHARD N. PODELL, M.D., M.P.H., Clinical Professor, Department of Family Medicine, UMDNJ-Robert Wood Johnson Medical School, and co-author of *The G-Index Diet: The Missing Link That Makes Permanent Weight Loss Possible*

"The glycemic index is a useful tool which may have a broad spectrum of applications, from the maintenance of fuel supply during exercise to the control of blood glucose levels in diabetics. Low glycemic index foods may prove to have beneficial health effects for all of us in the long term. *The Glucose Revolution* is a user-friendly, easy-to-read overview of all that you need to know about the glycemic index. This book represents a balanced account of the importance of the glycemic index based on sound scientific evidence."

—JAMES HILL, PH.D., Director, Center for Human Nutrition, University of Colorado Health Sciences Center

"*The New Glucose Revolution* summarizes much of the recent development of dietary glycemic index and load in a highly readable format. The authors are able researchers and respected leaders in the nutrition field. Much that is discussed in this book draws directly from their years of experimental and observational research. The focus on dietary intervention and prevention strategies in everyday eating is an especially laudable feature of this book. I recommend this book most highly as an indispensable source of good nutrition."

—SIMIN LIU, M.D., SC.D., Assistant Professor, Department of Epidemiology, Harvard School of Public Health

■

"As a coach of elite amateur and professional athletes, I know how critical the glycemic index is to sports performance. *The New Glucose Revolution* provides the serious athlete with the basic tools necessary for getting the training table right."

—JOE FRIEL, coach, author, consultant

Other Glucose Revolution & New Glucose Revolution Titles

The New Glucose Revolution: The Authoritative Guide to the Glycemic Index—the Dietary Solution for Lifelong Health

The Glucose Revolution Life Plan

What Makes My Blood Glucose Go Up... And Down? And 101 Other Frequently Asked Questions about Your Blood Glucose Levels

The New Glucose Revolution Complete Guide to Glycemic Index Values

The New Glucose Revolution Pocket Guide to Diabetes

The New Glucose Revolution Pocket Guide to Losing Weight

The New Glucose Revolution Pocket Guide to Sugar and Energy

■

The Glucose Revolution Pocket Guide to Sports Nutrition

The Glucose Revolution Pocket Guide to Your Heart

The Glucose Revolution Pocket Guide to the Glycemic Index and Healthy Kids

The Glucose Revolution Pocket Guide to Children with Type 1 Diabetes

■

FORTHCOMING

The New Glucose Revolution Pocket Guide to the Metabolic Syndrome

The New Glucose Revolution Pocket Guide to Peak Performance

The New Glucose Revolution Pocket Guide to Healthy Kids

The New Glucose Revolution Pocket Guide to Childhood Diabetes

The NEW GLUCOSE Revolution

POCKET GUIDE TO THE

TOP 100 LOW GI FOODS

Jennie Brand-Miller, Ph.D.
Johanna Burani, M.S., R.D., C.D.E.
Kaye Foster-Powell, M. Nutr. & Diet.

Marlowe & Company
New York

THE NEW GLUCOSE REVOLUTION POCKET GUIDE TO THE
TOP 100 LOW GI FOODS

Copyright © 2003 Jennie Brand-Miller, Kaye Foster-Powell,
and Johanna Burani

Published by
Marlowe & Company
An Imprint of Avalon Publishing Group Incorporated
245 West 17th Street • 11th Floor
New York, NY 10011

This edition was published in somewhat different form in Australia in
2002 under the title *The New Glucose Top 100 Low GI Foods* by Hodder
Headline Australia Pty Limited. This edition is published by arrange-
ment with Hodder Headline Australia Pty Limited.

Library of Congress Cataloging-in-Publication Data
Brand Miller, Janette, 1952–
The new glucose revolution pocket guide to the top 100
low GI foods / by Jennie Brand-Miller, Johanna Burani,
and Kaye Foster-Powell.—[Rev. and updated ed.]
Completely rev. and updated edition of: The glucose revolution pocket
guide to the top 100 low glycemic foods / Jennie Brand Miller and
Kaye Foster-Powell. New York : Marlowe, 2000.
Includes bibliographical references and index.
ISBN 1-56924-500-2
1. Glycemic index—Handbooks, manuals, etc. I. Title: Pocket guide to
the top 100 low glycemic foods. II. Foster-Powell, Kaye. III. Wolever,
Thomas M. S. IV. Foster Powell, Kaye. Glucose revolution pocket guide
to the top 100 low GI foods. V. Title.
QP701.B733 2003
613.2'83—dc21   2003052722
9 8 7 6 5 4 3 2 1

Designed by Pauline Neuwirth, Neuwirth & Associates, Inc.

Printed in the United States of America
Distributed by Publishers Group West

CONTENTS

Preface   xi

Introduction   xiii

1. What Is the Glycemic Index?   1
2. Let's Talk Glycemic Load   11
3. Secrets to Low-GI Snacking   15
4. Your Low-GI Food Finder   18
5. The Top 100 Low-GI Foods   23
6. A to Z GI Values   135

For More Information   153

Glycemic Index Testing   155

Acknowledgments   156

About the Authors   157

PREFACE

THE NEW GLUCOSE REVOLUTION is the definitive, all-in-one guide to the glycemic index (GI). Now we have written this pocket guide to answer one of the questions we are asked most frequently: "What foods have the lowest glycemic index values?"

The New Glucose Revolution Pocket Guide to the Top 100 Low GI Foods makes it easier than ever to identify those foods that have the lowest GI values—and to enjoy them every day, at every meal—for better blood-sugar control, weight loss, heart health, peak athletic performance, and overall well-being.

This book offers more in-depth information about the top 100 low-GI foods than we had room to include in *The New Glucose Revolution*. But this book has been written to be read alongside *The New Glucose Revolution*, so in the event you haven't already consulted that book, please be sure to do so for a more comprehensive discussion of the glycemic index and all its uses.

INTRODUCTION

*L*OW-GI FOODS are your key to unlocking the benefits of the glucose revolution. In this handy A to Z guide we show you which common foods have low glycemic index (or low GI) values and can help you to achieve an optimum diet for health and well-being.

Low-GI foods are those foods that contain carbohydrates that break down slowly, gradually releasing glucose into the bloodstream. They have the lowest values on the glycemic index (which we abbreviate as GI).

Here, in a nutshell, is everything important to know about the glycemic index:

> ● it's a scientifically proven measure of how carbohydrates affect blood-glucose levels—how different kinds of carbohydrate impact the amount of energy you feel after you eat;

- it helps you choose the right amount and right type of carbohydrate for your health and energy needs;
- it provides an easy and effective way to control blood-glucose fluctuations, providing you with longer-lasting energy and lessening your hunger.

The carbohydrates in high-GI foods break down quickly and have a fast sugar release into your bloodstream, while the carbohydrates in low-GI foods break down slowly and release sugar into your bloodstream much more slowly.

Low-GI foods have many benefits: They help you control your weight and appetite; they make it easier to manage diabetes; they reduce your risk of heart disease; and because they are, for the most part, high in fiber and nutrients, they improve your overall health.

This book will show you how to include low-GI foods in your diet. Each food entry contains nutritional information as well as some handy serving hints; you'll be surprised at how easy it is to fill your diet with low-GI foods. You can use the low GI food finder on page 18 to locate a food and use the condensed tables at the back of the book to find the glycemic index values of other foods. For more detailed tables you can also consult *The New Glucose Revolution* or the *Complete Guide to Glycemic Index Values*.

IT'S A COMMON misconception that sugar serves as your body's source of fuel. Not so. *Carbohydrates* provide the ideal fuel your body needs; sugar is merely a food ingredient.

1

WHAT IS THE GLYCEMIC INDEX?

WORLDWIDE RESEARCH SINCE the early 1980s
has shown us that different carbohydrate foods
have dramatically different effects on blood glucose levels. Until very recently it was widely believed that com-
plex carbohydrates, such as rice and potato, were best
for us. They were thought to be slowly digested energy
foods that caused only a small rise in our blood-glucose
levels. Sugars and concentrated sweets, on the other
hand, have been seen as villains that cause rapid fluctuations in blood-glucose levels. The glycemic index
research has turned all these beliefs upside down and
changed the way we think about carbohydrates—it truly
is a revolution.

When scientists began to study the actual blood-
glucose responses to different foods in hundreds of people, they found that many starchy foods (bread, potatoes,
etc.) are digested and absorbed very quickly and that
many sugar-containing foods (such as ice cream and

some cakes and cookies) were actually absorbed quite slowly.

The glycemic index (or GI) was developed simply as a measure of carbohydrate quality—the extent to which the carbohydrates in different foods will raise blood-glucose levels. Carbohydrate foods that break down quickly during digestion have the highest GI values. The blood-glucose response is fast and high. In other words, the glucose in the bloodstream spikes. Conversely, foods that contain carbohydrates that break down slowly, releasing glucose gradually into the bloodstream, have low glycemic index values, and produce slower and smaller responses.

The substance that produces one of the greatest effects on blood-glucose levels is pure glucose itself. *Most* foods have less effect than glucose when fed in equal amounts of carbohydrate. The glycemic index value of pure glucose is set at 100 and every other food is ranked on a scale from 0 to 100 according to the actual effect on blood-glucose levels.

■

**A high GI value is 70 or more.
An intermediate GI value is 56–69.
A low GI value is 55 or less.**

■

Today we know the GI values of hundreds of different food items that have been tested following the standardized method. The most recent and comprehensive values, and more information about how we measure the glycemic index and its health benefits, can be found in our latest book, *The New Glucose Revolution*.

■

**The glycemic index describes the type of carbohydrate
in foods. Different types of carbohydrates raise your
blood-glucose levels at different rates.**

■

WHAT IS CARBOHYDRATE?

Carbohydrate is either the starchy part of foods such as
rice, bread, potatoes, and pasta or the essential ingredients that make foods taste sweet: the sugars in fruit and
honey, and the refined sugars in soft drinks and candy,
for example.

Carbohydrate mainly comes from plant foods, such as
grains, fruits, vegetables, and legumes (peas and beans).
Milk products also contain carbohydrate in the form of
milk sugar, or lactose. Lactose is the first carbohydrate
we ingest as infants; there's more lactose in human milk
than in any other mammal's milk. It provides almost half
the energy an infant consumes daily while breast-feeding.

In the general food supply, some foods contain a large
amount of carbohydrate (such as grains, potatoes, and
legumes) while other foods have a minimal carbohydrate
content (such as broccoli and salad greens). Foods that
are high in carbohydrate include:

- Grains, including rice, wheat, oats, barley, rye,
  and anything made from them (bread, pasta,
  noodles, flour, breakfast cereals).
- Fruits such as apples, bananas, grapes, peaches, and
  melons, whether fresh, frozen, canned, or dried.

- Starchy vegetables, such as potatoes, yams, sweet corn, taro, and sweet potato.
- Legumes, including baked beans, lentils, kidney beans, peas, and chickpeas.
- Dairy products, including yogurt, milk, and ice cream.

Sources of Carbohydrate

PERCENTAGE OF carbohydrate (grams per 3½ ounces of food) in food as eaten:

Apple	12%	Orange	8%
Baked beans	11%	Pasta	70%
Banana	21%	Pear	12%
Barley	61%	Peas	8%
Bread	47%	Plum	6%
Cookies	62%	Potato	15%
Corn	16%	Raisins	75%
Cornflakes	85%	Rice	79%
Flour	73%	Split peas	45%
Grapes	15%	Sugar	100%
Ice cream	22%	Sweet potato	17%
Milk	5%	Tapioca	85%
Oats	61%	Water cracker	71%

HOW YOU CAN BENEFIT FROM EATING LOW-GI FOODS

The slow digestion and gradual rise and fall in blood-glucose responses after eating a low-GI food or meal has benefits for many people. Most important, it helps control the amount of glucose circulating in the blood, which serves as a huge benefit not only for people with diabetes but also for healthy people. If blood-glucose levels are reduced, there's a corresponding reduction in circulating insulin, as well. Limiting blood levels of insulin helps to protect against heart disease, diabetes, and obesity.

So low-GI foods can benefit everyone! Low-GI foods:

- result in lower insulin levels, which makes fat easier to burn and less likely to be stored
- help to lower blood fats
- are more satisfying and reduce appetite
- reduce the risk of developing diabetes
- help people with diabetes better manage their dietary needs
- reduce the risk of developing heart disease
- help to sustain endurance exercise for longer
- improve overall health

These facts aren't exaggerations, hunches, or opinions, or based on preliminary findings. They are confirmed results of many studies published in prestigious journals around the world.

WHAT DETERMINES A FOOD'S GLYCEMIC INDEX VALUE?

For decades, scientists have been studying what gives one food a high GI value and another one a low GI value. We've summarized the results of their research in the following table, which looks at the factors that influence the glycemic index value of a food.

The key message is that the *physical state* of the starch in the food is by far the most important factor influencing the GI value. That's why the advances in food processing over the past two hundred years have had such a profound (and negative) effect on the overall glycemic index values of the food we eat.

Factors That Influence a Food's Glycemic Index Value

Factor	Mechanism	Food examples
Starch gelatinization	The less gelatinized (swollen) the starch, the slower the rate of digestion.	Low GI: Al dente pasta, brown rice High GI: Overcooked pasta, sticky rice
Physical entrapment	The fibrous coat around beans and seeds and plant cell walls act as physical barriers, slowing down access of digestive enzymes to the starch inside.	Low GI: Pumpernickel and grainy bread, legumes, and barley High GI: Bagels, cornflakes
High amylose to amylopectin ratio*	The more amylose a food contains, the less easily the starch is gelatinized and the slower its rate of digestion.	Low GI: Basmati rice, legumes High GI: Enriched wheat flour products
Particle size	The smaller the particle size, the easier it is for water and enzymes to penetrate (the surface area is relatively greater).	Low GI: Stone-ground 100% whole wheat breads and crackers High GI: Enriched wheat flour products
Viscosity of fiber	Viscous, soluble fibers increase the viscosity of the intestinal contents and this slows down the interaction between the starch and the enzymes. Finely milled whole wheat and rye flours have *fast* rates of digestion and absorption because the fiber is not very thick or sticky.	Low GI: Rolled oats, beans and lentils, apples, Metamucil® High GI: Rice Krispies, kaiser roll

* Amylose and amylopectin are two different types of starch. Both are found in foods, but the ratio varies.

Factor	Mechanism	Food examples
Sugar	Sugar breaks down into 50% glucose and 50% fructose. Starch, such as enriched wheat flour, breaks down into 100% glucose. Therefore, the presence of some sugar in a food can lower its GI value. Sugar also inhibits the swelling of starch molecules, which also lowers its GI value.	Low GI: Sponge cake, pound cake HIGH GI: Croissant, pancakes
Acidity	Acids in foods slow down stomach emptying, thereby slowing the rate at which the starch can be digested. Examples of commonly used acids are vinegar, lemon juice, lime juice, salad dressings, and brine (used in pickles).	Low GI: Sourdough breads, sourdough English muffins HIGH GI: Enriched wheat white breads, crackers
Fat	Fat slows down the rate of stomach emptying, thereby slowing the digestion of the starch.	Low GI: Chocolate or white cake from mix HIGH GI: Angel food cake

EATING LOW-GI FOODS

Reaping the benefits of low-GI foods is easy. It just means making a few substitutions such as those listed on pages 9 and 10. Ideally, aim to swap at least half the foods you eat from a high-GI to a low-GI type. Perhaps you could change the type of bread or breakfast cereal you eat and consume pasta or legumes in moderate amounts.

HOW CAN YOU CHANGE YOUR DIET?

Some of the most common foods that will help you eat a lower-GI diet include:

- grainy breads
- low-GI breakfast cereals
- more fruit
- yogurt
- lots of pasta, beans, and vegetables

Eating any of the foods we recommend in this book will help you to lower the overall glycemic index value of your diet, but it isn't necessary to eat these foods exclusively. A balanced diet consists of a variety of foods. So if you eat a low-GI food with a high-GI food you will end up with a moderate GI value. What does this mean? It means that your blood-glucose response will be moderate and so will your circulating insulin level. And as we already stated, lower circulating blood glucose and insulin are good things.

To help yourself include low-GI foods:

- become familiar with them (use this book)
- plan; prepare a shopping list; keep a readily available supply in your fridge and kitchen cabinets
- experiment with them (try new foods and select low-GI recipes you think you'll enjoy)

Two of our other books, *The New Glucose Revolution* and *The Life Plan,* contain many easy and delicious low-GI recipes.

Remember:

- You don't have to avoid all high-GI foods to eat a low-GI diet.
- You do need to include a low-GI food at every meal.
- If you're not already eating low-GI foods, you should exchange about half the carbohydrate choices in your day from high-GI to low-GI types.
- If the high-GI foods you choose are high in carbohydrate, eat them in smaller quantities to reduce their glycemic load.

SUBSTITUTING LOW-GI FOR HIGH-GI FOODS

Look at the type of carbohydrate foods you eat (see pp. 3–4 for a list of carbohydrate foods). Identify those that you eat most, since these have the greatest glycemic impact on your body. Consider the high-carbohydrate foods you consume at each meal and replace at least one of these with one low-GI food. If you substitute half the total carbohydrate from high-GI to low-GI foods, you'll significantly reduce your diet's overall glycemic index value.

Switch from *this* high-GI food	To *this* low-GI alternative
Bread, whole wheat or white	Breads such as stone-ground whole wheat, sourdough, sourdough rye, and whole-grain pumpernickel

Switch from *this* high-GI food	To *this* low-GI alternative
Processed breakfast cereal, such as Cheerios, cornflakes, Rice Chex	Unrefined cereal such as old-fashioned oats or low-GI processed cereal such as All-Bran™
Plain cookies and crackers; vanilla wafers, rice cakes, saltines	Cookies made with dried fruit and whole grains such as oats (oatmeal cookies or Fifty50 cookies)
Cakes and muffins; angel food cake, doughnuts, scones	These baked goods made with fruit, oats, and whole-grain flours, or look for recipes on whole-grain cereal boxes
Tropical fruits such as bananas, papaya, pineapple, watermelon, and lychee	Temperate-climate fruits such as apples, peaches, and citrus
Potato: mashed, French fries, baked	New potatoes, sweet potatoes
Rice: sticky Jasmine, arborio	Basmati, brown, or long-grain rice

◀ 2 ▶

LET'S TALK GLYCEMIC LOAD

*I*N ADDITION TO the GI values we provide in this book, we also include the glycemic load (GL) value for average-sized food portions. Taken together, a food's GI value and glycemic load provide you with all the information you need to choose a diet brimming with health-boosting foods.

GLYCEMIC LOAD 101

A food's glycemic load results from the GI value and carbohydrate per serving of food. When we eat a carbohydrate-containing meal, our blood glucose first rises, then falls. The extent to which glucose rises and remains high is critically important to our health and depends on two things: the *amount* of a carbohydrate in the meal and the *nature* (glycemic index value) of that carbohydrate. Both factors equally determine blood-glucose changes.

Researchers at Harvard University came up with a way of combining and describing these two factors with the term "glycemic load," which not only provides a measure of the level of glucose in the blood, but also the insulin demand produced by a normal serving of the food. Researchers measure GI values for fixed portions of foods containing a certain amount of carbohydrate (usually 50 grams). Then, as people eat different-sized portions of the same foods, we can work out the extent to which a certain portion of food will raise the blood-glucose level by calculating a glycemic load value for that amount of food.

To calculate glycemic load, multiply a food's GI value by the amount of carbohydrate in a particular serving size, then divide by 100.

■

Glycemic load = (GI x carbohydrate per serving) ÷ 100

■

For example, a small apple has a GI value of 40 and contains 15 grams of carbohydrate. Its glycemic load is (40 x 15) ÷ 100 = 6. A small 5-ounce potato has a GI value of 90 and 15 grams of carbohydrate. It has a glycemic load of (90 x 15) ÷ 100 = 14. This means one small potato will raise your blood-glucose level higher than one apple.

Some nutritionists argue that the glycemic load is an improvement on the glycemic index because it provides an estimate of both quantity *and* quality of carbohydrate (the glycemic index gives us just quality) in a diet. In large Harvard studies, however, researchers were able to predict disease risk from people's overall diet, as well as its glycemic load. Using the glycemic load strengthened

How GI Values Affect Glycemic Load

THE GLYCEMIC LOAD is greatest for those foods that provide the highest-GI carbohydrate, particularly those we tend to eat in large quantities. Compare the glycemic load of the following foods to see how the serving size, as well as the GI value, helps to determine the glycemic response:

Rice, 1 cup	Spaghetti, 1 cup
Carbohydrates: 43	Carbohydrates: 40
GI: 83	GI: 44
GL: 36	GL: 18
$(83 \times 43) \div 100 = 36$	$(44 \times 40) \div 100 = 18$

the relationship, suggesting that the more frequently we consume high-carbohydrate, high-GI foods, the worse it is for our health. Carbohydrate by itself has no effect—in other words, there was no benefit to low carbohydrate intake over high carbohydrate intake, or vice versa.

■

Low GL = 10 or less
Intermediate GL = 11–19
High GL = 20 or more

■

If you make the mistake of using the GL alone, you might find yourself eating a diet with very little

carbohydrate but a lot of fat and excessive amounts of
protein. That's why you need to use the glycemic index
to compare foods of similar nature (such as bread with
bread) and use the glycemic load when you're deciding
on the portion size of the carbohydrates you want to eat.
If you use the technique correctly, GL values will guide
you to eat smaller portions of high-GI foods.

Remember that the GL values we provide are for the
standardized (nominal) portion sizes listed. If you eat a
different portion size, then you'll need to calculate
another GI value. Here's how: First, determine the
size of your portion, then work out the available carbohydrate content of this weight (this value is listed next to
the GL), then multiply by the food's GI value. For example, the nominal serving size listed for bran flakes is ½
cup, the available carbohydrate is 18 grams and the
glycemic index value is 74. So the GL for ½-cup serving
of bran flakes is (74 x 18) ÷ 100 = 13. If, however, you
normally eat 1 cup of bran flakes, you'd need to double
the available carbohydrate (18 x 2 = 36) and the GL for
your larger cereal portion would be (74 x 36) ÷ 100 = 27.
These numbers show that the larger portion of cereal
releases a larger quantity of glucose into the bloodstream.

◀ 3 ▶

SECRETS TO LOW-GI
SNACKING

*B*EFORE WE RUN down the Top 100 foods for you, this
might be a good time to talk about snacking. The fact
is, low-GI eating isn't limited to mealtime: It's normal to
get hungry and want to snack between your usual "three
squares." Luckily, when you eat the low-GI way there's no
prohibition on between-meal nibbles. (It's important to
remember that when you choose a snack, the glycemic
index value isn't all that matters; for added health benefits,
you should choose a snack that's low in fat, too.)

New evidence suggests that people who graze, eating
small amounts of food throughout the day at frequent
intervals, may actually be doing themselves a favor.
Spreading the food out over longer periods of time will
flatten out the peaks and valleys of blood-glucose levels.

. . .

ARE YOU REALLY CHOOSING LOW-FAT?

There's a trick to food labels that it is worth being aware of when shopping for low-fat foods. These food-labeling specifications guidelines were enacted by the United States Department of Agriculture (USDA) in 1994:

Free: Contains a tiny or insignificant amount of fat, cholesterol, sodium, sugar, or calories: less than 0.5 grams (g) of fat per serving.

Low-fat: Contains no more than 3 g of fat per serving.

Reduced/Less/Fewer: These diet products must contain 25 percent less of a nutrient to calories than the regular product.

Light/Lite: These diet products contain ⅓ fewer calories than, or ½ the fat of, the original product.

Lean: Meats with "lean" on the label contain less than 10 g of fat, 4 g of saturated fat, and 95 milligrams (mg) of cholesterol per serving.

Extra lean: These meats have less than 5 g of fat, 2 g of saturated fat, and 95 mg of cholesterol per serving.

17 Sustaining Snacks

- An apple
- An apple-and-oat-bran muffin
- Dried apricots
- A mini can of baked beans
- A small bowl of cherries
- Ice cream (low-fat) in a cone
- Milk, milkshake, or smoothie (low-fat, of course)
- Oatmeal cookies, 2 to 3
- An orange

- 6 ounces of orange juice, freshly squeezed
- Pita bread spread with apple butter
- A big bowl of low-fat popcorn
- 1 or 2 slices of raisin toast
- Whole-grain-bread sandwich with your favorite filling
- A bowl of oatmeal
- A small box of raisins
- 6 to 8 ounces of light yogurt

6 Snacking Tips

1. It's important to include a couple of servings of dairy foods each day to meet your calcium needs. If you haven't used yogurt or cheese in any meals, you may choose to make a low-fat milkshake. One or 2 scoops of low-fat ice cream or pudding can also boost your daily calcium intake.

2. If you like whole-grain breads, an extra slice makes a very good choice for a snack. Other snacks can include toasted sourdough English-muffin halves, a waffle, or a slice of raisin bread with a little butter.

3. Fruit is always a low-calorie option for snacks. You should try to consume at least 3 servings a day. It may be helpful to prepare fruit in advance to make it accessible and easy to eat.

4. Ryvita® whole-grain crispbreads are a low-calorie snack if you want something dry and crunchy.

5. Popcorn is another crunchy snack choice.

6. Keep vegetables (such as celery and carrot sticks, baby tomatoes, florets of blanched cauliflower, or broccoli) prepared and ready to serve.

◀ 4 ▶

YOUR LOW-GI FOOD FINDER

A high GI value is 70 or more.
An intermediate GI value is 56 to 69 inclusive.
A low GI value is 55 or less.

	◀	GI VALUE	▶			PAGE
	11-20	21-30	31-40	41-50	51-55	
	11-20					
Peanut Butter	14					100
Peanuts	14					101
Soybeans	14					118
Yogurt	14					134
Fructose	19					60
Maple Syrup	19					83
Rice Bran	19					112

	11-20	21-30	31-40	41-50	51-55	PAGE
		← GI VALUE →				
21-30						
Cashews		22				47
Cherries		22				49
Choice DM™ Beverage, Mead Johnson		23				54
Kidney Beans		23				72
Barley		25				33
Grapefruit		25				64
Lentils		26				77
Apples, Dried		29				29
Prunes, Dried		29				109
Black Beans		30				34
Hearty Oatmeal Cookies		30				68
31-40						
Apricots, Dried			31			31
Butter Beans			31			44
Chocolate, Milk, Sugar Free, Fifty50			31			52
Soy Milk			31			119
Lima Beans			32			78
Milk, Skim			32			85
Spaghetti, Whole Wheat			32			122
Split Peas, Dried			32			123
M&M's™ Peanut			33			80
Nutella®			33			89
Milk, Lowfat Chocolate			34			84
Hearty Chocolate Meal Replacement Drink			35			67
Ice Cream, Lowfat			37			70
Yam			37			133
All-Bran®			38			25

	11-20	21-30	31-40	41-50	51-55	PAGE
Cannellini Beans			38			45
Navy Beans			38			88
Pastina			38			97
Peaches, Canned			38			98
Pears			38			103
Rice, Converted			38			114
Tomato Juice			38			129
Tomato Soup			38			130
Mung Beans			39			87
Plums			39			106
Ravioli			39			111
Apple Juice			40			28
Apples			40			30
Fettuccine, Egg			40			59
Strawberries			40			125

	41-50	PAGE
Bread, Pumpernickel	41	38
Crème Filled Wafers, Vanilla	41	56
Blackeyed Peas	42	35
Chickpeas	42	50
Peaches	42	99
Spaghetti, Durum Wheat	42	121
Chocolate, Milk	43	51
Custard	43	57
Pudding	43	110
Lentil Soup	44	76
Capellini	45	46
Pinto Beans	45	105
Corn	46	55

	11-20	21-30	31-40	41-50	51-55	PAGE
		GI VALUE				
Grapes				46		66
Lactose				46		74
Sponge Cake				46		124
All-Bran Bran Buds				47		26
Macaroni				47		81
Baked Beans				48		32
Bulgur				48		43
Grapefruit Juice				48		65
Orange Marmalade				48		94
Oranges				48		95
Peas, Green				48		104
Sweet Potato				48		128
Pears, Canned				49		102
Muesli				49		86
Oat Bran Breakfast Cereal				50		90
Rice, Brown				50		113
Tortellini, Cheese, Frozen				50		131

	51-55	PAGE
All Bran with Extra Fiber	51	27
Bread, 100% Whole Grain	51	37
Mangoes	51	82
Oatmeal, Old-Fashioned	51	93
Strawberry Jam	51	126
Kidney Beans, Canned	52	71
Linguine, Thick	52	79
Spaghetti with Meat Sauce	52	120
Sushi	52	127
Bread, Sourdough Rye	53	39
Bread, Stoneground 100% Whole Wheat	53	41
Kiwi, Fresh	53	73

	◄══ GI VALUE ══►				PAGE
	11-20	21-30	31-40	41-50	51-55
Bread, Sourdough Wheat					54	40
Buckwheat					54	42
Oatmeal Cookies					54	92
Pound Cake					54	108
Rice, Long Grain and Wild					54	115
Fruit Cocktail					55	62
Honey					55	69
Oat Bran, Raw					55	91
Semolina					55	116
Social Tea Biscuits					55	117

◀ 5 ▶

THE TOP 100
LOW-GI FOODS

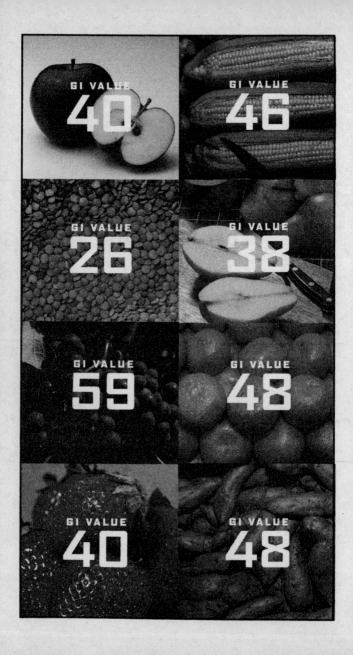

All-Bran®

(KELLOGG'S)

■

GI Value	**38**
Glycemic Load	**5**

Carbohydrate	13 g
Fat	1 g
Fiber	10 g

Serving size • ½ cup (1 oz)

A good source of B-group vitamins and excellent source of insoluble fiber, All-Bran® is made from coarsely milled wheat bran that has large pieces of endosperm (starch) still attached. The starch in All-Bran® is slowly broken down by the digestive enzymes in the small intestine. The large pieces of bran form a physical barrier to enzymatic attack while the large pieces of endosperm have a tightly packed, compact structure that is also resistant to digestion.

All-Bran® has a malty taste and is good topped with sliced banana or canned pear slices and milk. Or try sprinkling a few tablespoons over low-fat yogurt to help meet your daily fiber requirement. All-Bran® can also be added to muffins to make a hearty and satisfying low-GI treat.

All-Bran Bran Buds™

(KELLOGG'S)

■

GI Value	47
Glycemic Load	6

Carbohydrate	12 g
Fat	1 g
Fiber	12 g

Serving size • ⅓ cup (1 oz)

Along with All-Bran with Extra Fiber™, All-Bran Bran Buds™ is among the most fiber-rich breakfast cereals on the market. The sources of fiber come from wheat, corn bran, and psyllium (a soluble fiber that helps to reduce the risk of heart disease). This is a low-GI food that, because it is digested so slowly, keeps you feeling full for hours. Combine it with skim or 1% milk and fresh or unsweetened canned fruit for a great start in the morning.

All-Bran with Extra Fiber ™

(KELLOGG'S)

∎

GI Value	**51**
Glycemic Load	**5**

Carbohydrate	9 g
Fat	<1 g
Fiber	13 g

Serving size • ½ cup (.9 oz)

This cereal is a good source of B vitamins, as well as an excellent source of insoluble fiber. All-Bran is made from coarsely milled wheat bran that has large pieces of endosperm (starch) still attached. This minimizes the swelling of the starch molecules and limits the action of the digestive enzymes. All-Bran with Extra Fiber™ has a malty taste and is good topped with fresh or unsweetened canned fruit slices and milk. Alternatively, sprinkle a few tablespoons over a lower-fiber cereal to help meet your daily fiber requirement. You can also add All-Bran with Extra Fiber™ to muffins to boost the fiber content and lower the GI value of the finished product.

Apple Juice, Unsweetened

■

GI Value	40
Glycemic Load	12

Carbohydrate	29 g
Fat	0 g
Fiber	0 g

Serving size • 1 cup (8 oz)

Apple juice has a low GI value because of its high fructose content. Apples in all forms—and colors—contain potassium and vitamin C. Apple juice has some diuretic and laxative properties and aids in the overall functioning of the digestive system.

Apples, Dried

■

GI Value	**29**
Glycemic Load	**10**

Carbohydrate	34 g
Fat	0 g
Fiber	6 g

Serving size • 10 rings

Dried fruits, such as dried apples, are gaining in popularity with consumers. They are a convenient, portable, and healthy snack food, and are tasty ingredients in granolas, trail mixes, and baked fruit bars and desserts. They are available with or without added sugar, sulfured or unsulfured, and even in organic varieties. The nutritive value of dried apples is obviously elevated in comparison to the fresh fruit when compared by weight. So even just a few dried apple rings can provide lots of vitamins and minerals to your diet. Dried apples are a good source of potassium, vitamin C, and soluble and insoluble fiber.

Apples, Fresh

■

GI Value	**40**
Glycemic Load	**6**

Carbohydrate	16 g
Fat	0 g
Fiber	4 g

Serving size • 1 medium (about 4 oz)

Apples provide a crunchy, portable low-GI snack that's also a good source of fiber. Half the sugar in apples is fructose, which has a very low GI value. Fructose is more slowly absorbed than glucose and is only gradually converted to glucose in the liver. Apples are also high in malic acid (all acids slow down stomach emptying) and pectin (a soluble and viscous fiber that slows down the digestive process by increasing the viscosity of the intestinal contents). All of these factors act together to make apples a low-GI food. Cooking apples is likely to raise the GI value slightly because it breaks down the cell wall.

Apricots, Dried

■

GI Value	31
Glycemic Load	9

Carbohydrate	28 g
Fat	0 g
Fiber	5 g

Serving size • 17 halves

Dried apricots provide an excellent source of fiber and beta-carotene (the plant precursor of vitamin A) and are also a source of iron. This dried fruit makes a nourishing snack or addition to a school lunch box. The chewy, compact structure of dried apricots probably limits access by digestive juices and explains the reduction in their GI value compared with fresh apricots. Half the sugars are in the form of fructose, which produces very little effect on blood-sugar levels.

Baked Beans

■

GI Value	48
Glycemic Load	7

Carbohydrate	15 g
Fat	1 g
Fiber	7 g

Serving size • ½ cup

Canned baked beans are a popular, ready-to-eat form of legumes. The digestibility of legumes is determined primarily by the nature of the starch that is trapped in fibrous, thick-walled cells, which prevents the starch from swelling during cooking, slowing down its digestibility. Baked beans are commonly made from navy beans, which (like all legumes) have a high concentration of amylose. Canned baked beans make a good low-GI choice and are a healthy addition to any meal.

Barley, Pearled

•

GI Value	25
Glycemic Load	5

Carbohydrate	20 g
Fat	1 g
Fiber	3 g

Serving size • ½ cup cooked

*P*earled barley, a popular form of this cereal grain, has had the outer brown layers of husk removed. It is very nutritious and high in fiber, with one of the lowest GI values of any food. Much of the fiber is a viscous, soluble fiber, which helps to reduce the post-meal rise in blood glucose. It does this by slowing down the movement of the partially digested food through the small intestine, which slows down digestion. The near-intact structure of the grain also keeps the glycemic index value low. Use it in place of rice as a side dish or add it to soups, salads, casseroles, and stews.

Black Beans

■

GI Value	30
Glycemic Load	6

Carbohydrate	20 g
Fat	1 g
Fiber	11 g

Serving size • ¾ cup cooked

The black bean is a completely black kidney-shaped small bean used most often in Mexican cooking. It can also be added to soups, salads, and wraps for extra flavor and texture. As with other legumes, the black bean is a high-fiber food that our bodies digest slowly, permitting sustained feelings of fullness for several hours.

Black-eyed Peas

GI Value	42
Glycemic Load	10

Carbohydrate	24 g
Fat	1 g
Fiber	5 g

Serving size • ½ cup cooked

Also known as cowpeas and Southern peas, these are a small, kidney-shaped, cream-colored bean with a distinctive black "eye" and a subtle sweet flavor. Use them for soups and stews and in bean salads, or puree them. These peas are a traditional accompaniment to pork in the southern United States. They are an excellent source of folic acid, magnesium, and potassium, and a good source of iron, phosphorus, and certain B vitamins. They should be cooked for about an hour; if you overcook them, they will turn mushy. Black-eyed peas cause a small glucose rise because of the relatively slow or incomplete breakdown of their starch, which is mainly due to containment of the starch in intact cell walls and by its relatively high amylose content. The presence of phenolic compounds (such as tannins and catechins) in legumes tends to slow down digestion by inhibiting the action of the amylase enzymes.

Bread

ONE OF THE most important changes you can make to dramatically lower the GI value of your overall diet is to choose low-GI breads. Choose heavy grain breads, such as the brands listed in this book, instead of the refined white, brown, and whole-wheat breads. A general rule of thumb: The less processed, the coarser, and the denser a bread is, and the more fiber it contains, the lower the GI value. Stone-ground whole-wheat breads and white sourdough breads have lower GI values than conventional breads.

Bread, 100% Whole Grain™

(NATURAL OVENS)

■

GI Value	**51**
Glycemic Load	**7**

Carbohydrate	13 g
Fat	<1 g
Fiber	5 g

Serving size • 1 slice (1 oz)

*O*ne of Natural Ovens's highest-fiber breads, this loaf boasts 5 grams of fiber per slice; it's whole-grain and low in fat. Natural Ovens uses stone-ground whole-wheat flour, which produces larger carbohydrate particle sizes (whereas high-GI white bread has very small, easily digested carbohydrate particles). This bread also contains oats, a source of soluble fiber, and is fortified with lots of additional fiber, too. Natural Ovens breads are available in the United States by mail order. For ordering information, see page 153.

Bread, Pumpernickel

■

GI Value	41
Glycemic Load	5

Carbohydrate	12 g
Fat	<1 g
Fiber	3 g

Serving size • 1 slice (1 oz)

Also known as rye kernel bread, pumpernickel contains 80 to 90 percent whole and cracked rye kernels. It has a strong flavor and is dense and compact—not "airy" like some bread. Pumpernickel is usually sold thinly sliced. The main reason for its low GI value is its content of whole cereal grains. (Bread made from whole-wheat grains would be expected to have a similarly low GI value.)

Bread, Sourdough Rye

■

GI Value	53
Glycemic Load	6

Carbohydrate	12 g
Fat	<1 g
Fiber	1 g

Serving size • 1 slice (1 oz)

A buildup of organic acids gives sourdough bread its characteristic sour taste. This flavorful low-GI bread is a popular choice for takeout sandwiches to the office or for picnics or travel, because its compact structure keeps the sandwich intact. And the sour flavor blends well with a wide variety of meat, poultry, fish, and vegetable sandwich fillers.

Bread, Sourdough Wheat

■

GI Value	**54**
Glycemic Load	**8**

Carbohydrate	14 g
Fat	<1 g
Fiber	1 g

Serving size • 1 slice (1 oz)

Sourdough results from the deliberately slow fermentation of flour by yeast, which produces a buildup of organic acids. These acids give the bread its characteristic sour taste. Once eaten, sourdough bread is slowly released from the stomach into the small intestine, where the body digests it. The slower the rate of "gastric emptying" and the slower release of glucose into the blood gives sourdough breads low GI values.

Bread, Stone-ground 100% Whole-Wheat

■

GI Value	53
Glycemic Load	7

Carbohydrate	13 g
Fat	1 g
Fiber	2 g

Serving size • 1 slice (1 oz)

"Stone-ground 100% whole-wheat bread" means that the flour used has been milled from the entire wheat berry (the germ, endosperm or starch compartment, and the bran) and that the milling process used is a method of slowly grinding the grain with a burrstone instead of metal rollers to more evenly distribute the germ oil. Virtually none of the ingredients packaged in the wheat berry get lost in this processing method. That's why this bread is a rich source of several B vitamins, iron, zinc, and dietary fiber.

Buckwheat

■

GI Value	**54**
Glycemic Load	**16**

Carbohydrate	30 g
Fat	1 g
Fiber	4 g

Serving size • ¾ cup cooked groats

Buckwheat grains must be hulled to be edible. The cracked whole buckwheat "groats" (also known as kasha) that result from hulling can be roasted and used just like rice or potatoes in soups, pilafs, or stews, or as a cooked cereal. The intact whole seed structure accounts for the low GI value because the seed coat limits access of digestive enzymes.

Buckwheat flour is also used in pancakes, muffins, cookies, and cakes and to make Russian *blinis* and Japanese *soba* noodles. In any form, buckwheat provides potassium, magnesium, zinc, iron, calcium, copper, soluble fiber, and several B vitamins.

Bulgur (Cracked Wheat)

■

GI Value	48
Glycemic Load	11

Carbohydrate	23 g
Fat	0 g
Fiber	6 g

Serving size • ½ cup cooked

Bulgur is made by coarsely grinding dried cooked wheat grains. The parboiling and light crushing of the wheat grain in the process of making bulgur has only a small effect on its GI value. Bulgur is prevalent in Middle Eastern cuisine. Tabouli, the popular Lebanese salad, consists of a mixture of parsley, bulgur, chopped tomato, onion, and dressing. The compactness and intact physical form of the wheat contribute to its low GI value.

Butter Beans

•

GI Value	31
Glycemic Load	4

Carbohydrate	15 g
Fat	0 g
Fiber	5 g

Serving size • ½ cup cooked

The slow digestibility of all legumes (including butter beans) is determined by the nature of the starch that's entrapped in fibrous, thick-walled cells. This prevents the starch from swelling during cooking and reducing its digestibility.

Butter beans are delicious in soups. You can add the canned variety to summer salads. These beans are rich in B vitamins, especially heart-healthy folic acid, minerals, and fiber.

Cannellini Beans, Canned

∎

GI Value	38
Glycemic Load	4

Carbohydrate	11 g
Fat	1 g
Fiber	8 g

Serving size • ½ cup cooked beans

Also known as white kidney beans, cannellini beans are large, elongated, kidney-shaped beans with a white, cream-colored skin. Like all legumes, these beans have a low GI value. It takes a relatively long time for digestive enzymes to penetrate the bean's external seed coat to reach the encapsulated starch molecules that will become the glucose that's released into your bloodstream. These beans accent soups, stews, and salads, and blend well with tomatoes, or with fresh herbs such as thyme, rosemary, mint, oregano, and marjoram, or with spices such as cardamom and nutmeg. Cannellini beans are filled with vitamins and minerals, most notably folic acid and potassium. They're also an excellent source of fiber, especially the heart-healthy insoluble form. Though dried beans are nutritionally denser, the canned version is a fine second choice for its convenience and versatility.

Cappellini Pasta

■

GI Value	**45**
Glycemic Load	**20**

Carbohydrate	45 g
Fat	1 g
Fiber	2 g

Serving size • 1 cup cooked

*C*appellini is the thinnest form of pasta made from the durum (hard) wheat form, semolina. This high-gluten flour gives all forms of pasta made from it a dense consistency, which slows the breakdown of its starch molecules. This slow breakdown produces a slow release of glucose into the bloodstream and a low glycemic index value. Because cappellini is so thin, it's easy to overcook. Optimal cooking time is four minutes for a perfect al dente product. This type of pasta tastes best with light, smooth, or spicy sauces, such as tomato, marinara, or pesto.

NOTE: Don't mistake cappellini for angel-hair pasta, another form of very long, thin pasta. Although angel-hair pasta is similar in shape to cappellini, its dough is made with eggs.

Cashews

∎

GI Value	**22**
Glycemic Load	**3**

Carbohydrate	13 g
Fat	23 g
Fiber	2 g

Serving size • approx. 32 nuts

Cashews, like all other nuts, are cholesterol free and high in protein. Their carbohydrate content is very low, which accounts for their low GI value. Cashews have a high fat content (almost half of their total weight), but they contain less fat than any other type of nut. Three-quarters of the fat in cashews is the heart-healthy poly-unsaturated kind, primarily monounsaturated; they're also rich in several B vitamins and a variety of minerals, most notably copper, magnesium, and zinc. Cashews are a healthy addition to salads, rice dishes, and desserts, and are a common ingredient in Asian dishes. They can even be ground into a creamy butter that you can use in place of peanut butter. Because of their high nutrient content and high caloric density, it's best to eat cashews several times a week, but in small amounts.

Cereal Grains

IN EARLY TIMES, grain preparation involved rough grinding between stones, breaking the outer seed husk but leaving much of the grain intact. This limited gelatinization of the starch during cooking and reduced the rate of digestion. The presence of anti-nutrients (such as phytic acid), which occur naturally in cereal grains, further limited digestion. Today, cereal processing includes milling to a fine flour, popping, toasting, flaking, and extrusion cooking to make products such as cakes, breads, biscuits, snack products, and breakfast cereals. The processing makes the starch readily digested and the GI value high.

Cherries, Fresh

■

GI Value	**22**
Glycemic Load	**1**

Carbohydrate	5 g
Fat	0 g
Fiber	1 g

Serving size • 10 cherries

Cherries are a good source of potassium and vitamin C and have the lowest GI value of any fruit scientists have examined so far. We don't know exactly why the cherry's GI value is so low, but this fruit does have a somewhat rubbery consistency, just like pasta and dried apricots, which is known to increase resistance to disruption in the intestine. Cherries are also acidic and high in sugars, both of which slow down the rate of stomach emptying (and therefore digestion). Canned cherries in heavy syrup are likely to have a higher GI value. This fruit must be picked ripe since it won't ripen after harvesting.

Chickpeas (Garbanzo Beans), Canned

GI Value	**42**
Glycemic Load	**9**

Carbohydrate	22 g
Fat	1 g
Fiber	5 g

Serving size • ½ cup

Also known as garbanzo beans, chickpeas are the main ingredient in such Middle Eastern specialties as hummus (a cold spreadable puree) and falafel (fried balls or patties). Roasted chickpeas, sprinkled with salt and spices, make a healthy low-GI snack. The low glycemic index value of chickpeas is due to the encapsulation of the starch in a hard seed coat, a higher amylose ration in the starch, and the presence of tannins and enzyme inhibitors that slow down digestion. And although canned chickpeas have a slightly higher GI value than the boil-at-home version, they are a quick way for vegetarians (and others) to get a low-GI source of protein. Canned chickpeas are especially convenient to pop into salads and pita sandwiches for a quick, nutritious, low-GI lunch.

Chocolate, Milk

■

GI Value	43
Glycemic Load	8

Carbohydrate	19 g
Fat	8 g
Fiber	0 g

Serving size • 1 oz

*M*ost people are surprised to learn that the world's favorite food has a relatively low glycemic index value. Although half the weight is sugar, fat contributes most of the calories in chocolate. This much fat slows down stomach emptying so that the sugar reaches the small intestine gradually, and produces only a moderate rise in blood-glucose levels, accounting for its low GI value.

Because chocolate is calorically dense, allow for a small indulgence every once in a while—then you can enjoy its wonderful taste, without the guilt!

Children and Low-fat Diets

Young children (under age five) rely on a certain amount of fat in their diet as a source of calories and should generally not be placed on a low-fat diet. A moderate amount of fat is also necessary as a source of essential fatty acids and fat-soluble vitamins.

Chocolate, Milk, Sugar Free

(FIFTY50)

■

GI Value	31
Glycemic Load	7

Carbohydrate	21 g
Fat	14 g
Fiber	<1 g

Serving size • 7 sections

This smooth, rich-tasting chocolate is a perfect palate-pleasing treat for anyone intent on controlling blood-sugar levels. Its low-GI value is a direct result of the low-GI sweeteners and fats formulated to produce a thick, creamy texture and sweet taste. Like any dietary "extra," these milk-chocolate calories should be planned into your balanced diet.

Chocolate, the Mood Food: Can It Be Good for Your Health?

DID YOU EVER think of chocolate as being a plant-based food? Well, it is. Chocolate is made from the cocoa bean, which grows on cacao trees in the rain forests of South America and Africa. Chocolate contains phosphorus, potassium, and iron, as well as flavonoids. Flavonoids, naturally occurring phytochemicals, have antioxidant properties that protect against some forms of cancer and heart disease. Chocolate also contains a chemical called phenylethylamine, which works on your brain's neurotransmitters and produces a calming, somewhat euphoric effect. In fact, some people equate chocolate's effect on their mood with being in love!

Choice DM™ Beverage
(MEAD JOHNSON)

■

GI Value	**23**
Glycemic Load	**6**

Carbohydrate	21 g
Fat	10 g
Fiber	3 g

Serving size • 1 cup (8 oz)

This product is a nutritionally complete oral supplement designed for people with diabetes, glucose intolerance, or stress-induced hyperglycemia. While there are many similar products on the market, Choice is among the varieties with the lowest GI values. It's always best to nourish your body with whole, natural foods. However, for reasons that may warrant its use, temporarily or long-term, Choice is a healthy low-GI oral-supplement option.

Corn, Canned, No Salt Added

■

GI Value	**46**
Glycemic Load	**13**

Carbohydrate	28 g
Fat	1 g
Fiber	3 g

Serving size • 1 cup

Corn contains folic acid, potassium, the antioxidant vitamins A and C, and dietary fiber. Canned corn is used in soups, mixed vegetables, stews, relishes, and salads, and manufacturers use fresh corn to make tortillas, hominy grits, polenta, corn bread, cornflakes, and corn oil. Topped with just a hint of butter, corn makes an excellent starchy vegetable side dish.

Crème Filled Wafers, Vanilla

(FIFTY50)

■

GI Value	41
Glycemic Load	8

Carbohydrate	20 g
Fat	9 g
Fiber	<1 g

Serving size • 6 cookies

The wafer part of this cookie is sweetened with the non-nutritive sweetener aspartame and with the sugar alcohol sorbitol. (The crème filling also contains sorbitol.) The sorbitol helps to prolong the time it takes for the digested carbohydrate to enter your bloodstream as glucose, because it is slowly absorbed from the intestinal tract and must go to the liver to be metabolized.

Custard

■

GI Value	**43**
Glycemic Load	**10**

Carbohydrate	24 g
Fat	5 g
Fiber	0 g

Serving size • ¾ cup (whole milk)

Custard is prepared from commercial wheat starch with egg, milk, and sugar added. Its low GI value may be explained by its fat content (which slows down stomach emptying) and its sugars, sucrose and lactose, which have only half the glycemic effect of pure wheat starch. Custard makes a creamy, sweet, low-GI dessert. Sprinkle a little nutmeg on top for an old-fashioned look and taste.

Dairy Foods

LACTOSE IS THE sugar found naturally in milk and milk products and is one reason behind their low GI values (see "Lactose," page 74). The presence of protein, fat, and lactic acid in fermented milk products such as yogurt, cheese, and sour cream slows down stomach emptying and lowers the glycemic index value. Skim or lowfat milk, yogurt, ice cream, puddings, and custards are excellent sources of calcium with low GI values. Note: Cheese, although another source of calcium, is not a source of carbohydrate because the lactose is drawn off in the whey during cheese manufacturing.

Fettuccine, Egg

■

GI Value	40
Glycemic Load	18

Carbohydrate	46 g
Fat	1 g
Fiber	2 g

Serving size • 1 cup

Fettuccine is a ribbon-shaped pasta, about one-fifth of an inch wide. It's made from semolina and other ingredients such as spinach, tomato paste, and even cocoa. It tastes best with tomato-based or cheese-based sauces. All forms of pasta have a dense consistency, which makes this popular carbohydrate resistant to disruption in the small intestine and contributes to the final low GI value.

Fructose

■

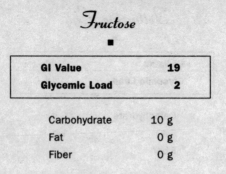

GI Value	**19**
Glycemic Load	**2**

Carbohydrate	10 g
Fat	0 g
Fiber	0 g

Serving size • 1 tablespoon

Fructose (or fruit sugar) is a form of sugar that occurs naturally in all fruits and in honey. Apples are a particularly rich source of free fructose. This sugar is slowly absorbed into the bloodstream and only gradually converted to glucose in the liver. Its presence in the liver brings about a prompt reduction in the body's normal glucose-producing mechanisms (something that glucose doesn't do). All in all, fructose has only 20 percent of the effect of pure glucose on blood-glucose and insulin levels. We must state, however, that very large amounts of fructose have undesirable effects on blood fats, specifically triglycerides. For this reason, it's best to derive fructose from fruits rather than from foods sweetened with high fructose corn syrup.

Avoid the Confusion

WHILE FRUCTOSE OCCURS naturally in fruit, honey, and even some vegetables, high fructose corn syrup (HFCS) is something very different. HFCS is a potent sweetener used in bakery and confectionary items and most often in soft drinks and many commercial varieties of fruit juices and drinks. In fact, HFCS in sodas currently contributes 33 percent of total U.S. sugar consumption. Made from cornstarch, it is sometimes poorly absorbed in the intestine, causing cramps, bloating, and diarrhea. There is accumulating scientific evidence that fructose may elevate blood triglycerides. The culprit doesn't appear to be the *natural* food sources of fructose, but rather the highly concentrated HFCS. The bottom line? Enjoy fresh fruits and vegetables and limit your consumption of baked goods and concentrated sweets, including soft drinks. Where have you heard that before?

Fruit Cocktail

■

GI Value	55
Glycemic Load	9

Carbohydrate	16 g
Fat	0 g
Fiber	1 g

Serving size • ½ cup

Fruit cocktail usually consists of a mixture of peaches, pears, seedless grapes, pineapple, and cherries—mostly low-GI fruit. The labels "natural," "lite/light," and "in real fruit juices" are all ways of saying that there has been no sugar added to canned fruit. See the box on the next page for more information about fruit.

Fruit

THE MAJORITY OF fruits are low-GI foods. The presence of sugars (especially fructose) with low GI values, fibers (both soluble and insoluble) and acids (which may slow down stomach emptying) are probable reasons. The fruits with the lowest GI values tend to be those grown in temperate climates, such as apples, peaches, pears, citrus, cherries, and berries. The more acidic the fruit, the lower the glycemic index value (e.g., grapefruit's GI is 25). Tropical fruits such as watermelon, pineapple, cantaloupe, and bananas have intermediate GI values.

All fresh fruits are a source of vitamin C; you should eat at least two to three servings every day. Refer to the Food Guide Pyramid for portion recommendations.

Grapefruit, Fresh

■

GI Value	**25**
Glycemic Load	**2**

Carbohydrate	11 g
Fat	0 g
Fiber	1 g

Serving size • ½ medium

Half a grapefruit contains about 42 mg of vitamin C, making it an excellent source for this antioxidant. It is high in citric acid, which lowers the GI value by slowing down stomach emptying. Grapefruit is a refreshing food to eat at breakfast, halved and eaten as is or sprinkled with a little sugar. It can also be peeled and segmented and included in fruit or vegetable salads.

Grapefruit Juice, Unsweetened

■

GI Value	**48**
Glycemic Load	**11**

Carbohydrate	22 g
Fat	0 g
Fiber	0 g

Serving size • 1 cup (8 oz)

*C*ool and refreshing after a workout or with breakfast, a glass of grapefruit juice provides not only liquid refreshment, but nutritional benefits as well. Rich in the antioxidant vitamin C, grapefruit juice is also high in citric acid, which slows down stomach emptying and lowers the juice's GI value. Many commercial brands now add extra calcium to grapefruit juice for a drink that's a powerhouse of antioxidant and bone-building protection. For a new taste sensation, try mixing grapefruit juice with club soda—the result is a tangy, fizzy beverage!

Grapes, Green
■

GI Value	**46**
Glycemic Load	**8**

Carbohydrate	18 g
Fat	0 g
Fiber	1 g

Serving size • approx. 17

Grapes have one of the highest sugar contents among temperate fruits. This is one reason they make a good starting ingredient for alcoholic beverages (more sugar means more alcohol). The high sugar content reduces the rate of stomach emptying, which slows down digestion and absorption. Grapes are also quite high in acid, another factor that slows down the rate of food entering the small intestine. They're the perfect snack food—convenient to carry and eat on the run. No mess! One caveat: This finger-food fruit adds up to a lot of carbs (glycemic load) if you eat too many at once. Consider one cup (or a handful) per serving.

Hearty Chocolate Meal Replacement Drink

(FIFTY50)

■

GI Value	**35**
Glycemic Load	**11**

Carbohydrate	32 g
Fat	4 g
Fiber	3 g

Serving size • 1 cup (8 oz)

This ready-to-mix meal-replacement powder is sweetened with fructose, which is a low-GI sugar. When made with low-fat milk, an 8-ounce glass of this drink qualifies as a healthy, quick, on-the-run meal, providing 210 calories and one-third of the recommended daily values for 19 essential vitamins and minerals.

Hearty Oatmeal Cookies
(FIFTY50)

■

GI Value	30
Glycemic Load	6

Carbohydrate	20 g
Fat	7 g
Fiber	1 g

Serving size • 4 cookies

These cookies are made with two ingredients that rank as low-GI foods: fructose (GI = 19), and rolled oats (GI = 55). The addition of a moderate amount of fat (7 grams in four cookies) also slows the breakdown of the cookie's carbohydrate as glucose. Low-GI sweets, such as these cookies, help round out any balanced diet.

Honey

■

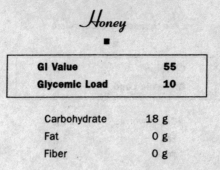

GI Value	55
Glycemic Load	10

Carbohydrate	18 g
Fat	0 g
Fiber	0 g

Serving size • 1 tablespoon

*H*oney is a concentrated source of carbohydrate and is basically a mixture of glucose and fructose. Honey's GI value appears to be similar to that of refined sugar (about 60), unless it is glucose enriched (which increases its glycemic index value). Honey was a major source of sweetness at the beginning of the nineteenth century— long before refined sugar became available. In fact, historical research suggests that in some parts of the world people ate quantities of honey similar to the amount of refined sugar we now eat. There are negligible quantities of other nutrients in honey.

Ice Cream, Low-fat

■

GI Value	**37**
Glycemic Load	**5**

Carbohydrate	14 g
Fat	3 g
Fiber	0 g

Serving size • ½ cup

*I*ce cream is a source of calcium. Look for low-fat or nonfat ice creams when you shop. Some taste as good as or better than their full-fat counterparts. Ice cream has a higher GI value than milk because of the presence of added sugar in addition to lactose. Small portions of this low-GI treat will help keep your glycemic load low.

Kidney Beans, Red, Canned

■

GI Value	52
Glycemic Load	6

Carbohydrate	12 g
Fat	<1 g
Fiber	6 g

Serving size • ½ cup

Although canned kidney beans have a higher GI value than home-boiled kidney beans, they still qualify as a low-GI food. The high temperatures and/or pressures of the canning process soften the seed casing and induce greater degrees of starch gelatinization in the beans' starch interior, which allows for quicker digestion. Nonetheless, canned kidney beans are a low-GI food, high in fiber, iron, B vitamins, and protein, and can make a valuable addition to your diet.

Kidney Beans, Red, Dried

■

GI Value	23
Glycemic Load	3

Carbohydrate	13 g
Fat	<1 g
Fiber	7 g

Serving size • ½ cup cooked

This is the type of bean used in vegetarian and meat chili, as well as in tacos and burritos. This nutrient-packed vegetable-protein food has been replaced by the more convenient canned form with relatively no nutritional loss. Traditionally, dried kidney beans are soaked overnight and can be boiled for two hours without losing their shape or texture. Not only are kidney beans a wonderful addition to Mexican and Tex-Mex cuisines, they make a great side dish for any meal. Like all other legumes, kidney beans have a low GI value because of their hard outer seed encasement and the low degree of gelatinization of their interior starch.

Kiwi, Fresh

•

GI Value	53
Glycemic Load	4

Carbohydrate	8 g
Fat	0 g
Fiber	3 g

Serving size • 1 average

The furry kiwi provides lots of the antioxidant vitamin C. This acidic fruit contains equal proportions of glucose (a high-GI sugar) and fructose (a low-GI sugar), which results in an intermediate GI value. Kiwis are also quite acidic; the acids slow down stomach emptying and result in slower rates of digestion and absorption in the small intestine. Enjoy versatile kiwis in salads, sandwiches, and desserts.

Lactose

◼

GI Value	46
Glycemic Load	5

Carbohydrate	10 g
Fat	0 g
Fiber	0 g

Serving size • 1 tablespoon

*L*actose is a disaccharide ("double sugar") that needs to be digested into its component sugars before the body can absorb it. The two sugars, glucose and galactose, compete with each other for absorption. Once absorbed, galactose is mainly metabolized in the liver, producing little effect on plasma glucose levels. The remaining sugar in lactose, glucose, is present in a small enough amount to prevent a spike in blood glucose.

Some people are lactose intolerant because the enzyme lactase is no longer active in their small intestine, but that should not stop them from enjoying lactose-reduced or lactose-free milk and milk products throughout the day. Lactose-intolerant people can usually tolerate yogurt because the microorganisms in the yogurt are active in digesting lactose during passage through the small intestine. Cheese is a good source of calcium, too, that is virtually free of lactose.

Legumes

LEGUMES (SUCH AS lentils, kidney beans, pinto beans, cannellini beans, dried peas, chickpeas, and soybeans) are nature's lowest-GI foods. The reasons include the encapsulation of the starch in a hard seed coat, a higher amylose ratio in the starch, and the presence of substances that slow down digestion, such as tannins and enzyme inhibitors, that are not destroyed in the cooking process. They also contain starch, which is totally resistant to digestion in the small intestine. Resistant starch behaves like fiber in the large bowel and may reduce the risk of developing colon cancer.

Legumes are rich in folic acid, potassium, magnesium, iron, and fiber. They're a great asset to a healthy diet. You can eat legumes hot or cold, straight from the can, or pureed. They can be ground into flour, and they can be roasted, fermented, or eaten as sprouts.

Lentil Soup, Canned

■

GI Value	**44**
Glycemic Load	**9**

Carbohydrate	21 g
Fat	1 g
Fiber	5 g

Serving size • 1 cup

*B*ecause of the high quality and caloric density of the nutrients in even commercially prepared lentil soup, it qualifies as a meal by itself. Just remember to choose a low-sodium product. The low GI value of lentil soup results from the same properties that all legumes share: encapsulated starch in the hard seed coat, a high quantity of amylose, and the presence of substances that slow digestion. For all of these reasons, the lentils in soup are very slowly broken down and very slowly released into the bloodstream.

Lentils, Brown, Dried

■

GI Value	**26**
Glycemic Load	**3**

Carbohydrate	12 g
Fat	0 g
Fiber	8 g

Serving size • ½ cup cooked

Lentils are rich in protein, fiber, and B vitamins. They are often used as substitutes for meat in vegetarian recipes. The red lentil is one of the oldest known beans. All colors and types of lentils have a similarly low GI value, which is increased slightly by canning. They have a fairly bland, earthy flavor and are best prepared with onion, garlic, and spices.

Lima Beans, Baby, Frozen

■

GI Value	**32**
Glycemic Load	**5**

Carbohydrate	17 g
Fat	0 g
Fiber	6 g

Serving size • ½ cup

All legumes, including the lima bean, have a low GI value. The lima bean is a larger variety of the butter bean. It has a floury texture and slightly sweet flavor. Baby lima beans can be boiled and served as a vegetable side dish. Dried and canned lima beans can also be used in soups, stews, casseroles, and salads. The reason legumes are nature's lowest-GI foods is because of the encapsulation of the starch in a hard seed coat, a higher amylose ratio in the starch and the presence of substances that slow down digestion—such as tannins and enzyme inhibitors—that aren't destroyed in the cooking process.

Linguine, Thick

■

GI Value	**52**
Glycemic Load	**23**

Carbohydrate	45 g
Fat	1 g
Fiber	2 g

Serving size • 1 cup cooked

Their name means "tongues," to represent this pasta's flat, slippery shape. This pasta is made from semolina, or durum (hard) wheat flour, with a high gluten content. Gluten is the protein portion of the wheat that forms a type of webbing around the starch molecules that slows their digestion into glucose. That means glucose is released into the bloodstream slowly, giving linguine a low GI value. Pesto and clam sauces serve as ideal sauces for linguine.

Low-GI Eating

THE EMPHASIS IS on whole, natural, minimally processed foods such as whole grains—barley, oats, dried peas and beans, breads, pasta, rice, vegetables, and fruits. Stock your pantry with these foods and keep a loaf of whole-grain bread in the freezer. For recipes, check out our books *The New Glucose Revolution* or *The Glucose Revolution Life Plan*, which include dozens of recipes specially modified to lower your diet's overall GI value, plus new ways of preparing low-GI foods.

M&M's™ (Peanut)

■

GI Value	**33**
Glycemic Load	**11**

Carbohydrate	33 g
Fat	10 g
Fiber	1 g

Serving size • 1 packet (1.69 oz)

M&M's™ milk chocolate candy with peanuts, with its low GI value, is an example of a "fun food" that you can work into a balanced diet without feeling guilty. The key is to keep the serving size small, because you get more enjoyment than nutrients from this low-GI snack. When you eat small amounts from small, individual-sized packages rather than handfuls from a one-pound bag, M&M's™ won't elevate your blood-sugar levels, your cholesterol, or even your weight!

Macaroni

■

GI Value	**47**
Glycemic Load	**18**

Carbohydrate	38 g
Fat	1 g
Fiber	2 g

Serving size • 1 cup cooked

*P*asta, in any size or shape, has a relatively low GI value (30 to 60). The reason for its slow digestion is the physical entrapment of the starch molecules in the sponge-like network of the protein (gluten) molecules in the pasta dough. This enclosure prevents the starch from swelling and consequently inhibits its breakdown into glucose and its entering the blood. In other words, like other low-GI foods, pasta doesn't elevate blood-sugar levels. This is good news for pasta lovers, who should still keep portion size in mind. If you eat too large a portion of even a low-GI food, the glucose load becomes too large and this will negatively affect your blood-sugar levels after you eat. A popular form of pasta, macaroni combines well with tomato- or other vegetable-based sauces.

Mangoes, Fresh
■

GI Value	51
Glycemic Load	10

Carbohydrate	19 g
Fat	0 g
Fiber	2 g

Serving size • ½ fruit (about 4 oz)

*M*angoes are one tropical fruit that squeezes into the low-GI range. Most tropical fruits have higher GI values than temperate fruit, possibly related to differences in acidity and sugar content. Rich in naturally occurring sugars, vitamin C, and vitamin A precursors, mangoes are also versatile: You can eat them in fruit salads and crepes and as a salsa base for fish, meat, poultry, and legumes. You can also enjoy them as is or with breakfast cereals. This fruit tastes best at peak ripeness.

Maple Syrup, Fructose Sweetened, Reduced Calorie

(FIFTY50)

■

GI Value	**19**
Glycemic Load	**3**

Carbohydrate	18 g
Fat	0 g
Fiber	0 g

Serving size • ¼ cup

The main ingredient in this maple-flavored table syrup is low-GI fructose (GI = 19), which is one of the naturally occurring sugars in fruit. Fructose, natural gums, and maple flavoring are combined in a water solution to produce a thick, syrupy consistency, an ideal topping for whole-grain pancakes, waffles, or French toast. Because this syrup contains calories, one-quarter cup is the recommended portion size.

Milk, Low-fat, Chocolate with Sugar

■

GI Value	34
Glycemic Load	9

Carbohydrate	26 g
Fat	3 g
Fiber	0 g

Serving size • 1 cup (8 oz)

Adding a moderate amount of refined sugar in the form of chocolate syrup or powder does not significantly raise the glycemic index value of 1% milk. For many young people (and adults as well) who don't care for the taste of plain milk or prefer something a bit sweeter, this is an excellent dairy choice that can help add some extra vitamins and minerals to the day's nutrient intake.

Milk, Skim

■

GI Value	**32**
Glycemic Load	**4**

Carbohydrate	13 g
Fat	0 g
Fiber	0 g

Serving size • 1 cup (8 oz)

This is the most nutritious form of milk for the least amount of calories (approximately 90). The GI value of skim milk is slightly higher than that of whole milk, because there is no fat to slow down the gastric emptying. But all forms of milk have low GI values. For people trying to cut fat in their diet, switching from whole or 2% milk to skim or 1% is a great first step.

Muesli, Natural

■

GI Value	49
Glycemic Load	10

Carbohydrate	20 g
Fat	3 g
Fiber	5 g

Serving size • 1 oz

Muesli originated as a Swiss health food and currently rates as one of the few relatively unprocessed breakfast cereals on the market. It is a good source of thiamin, riboflavin, and niacin. The low glycemic index value results because the oats are eaten raw, and are therefore in an ungelatinized state that resists digestion in the small intestine. Oats also contain a fiber that increases the viscosity of the contents of the small intestine, thereby slowing down the "enzyme attack." This same fiber has also been shown to reduce blood-cholesterol levels.

Mung Beans, Cooked

■

GI Value	**39**
Glycemic Load	**9**

Carbohydrate	23 g
Fat	<1 g
Fiber	15 g

Serving size • 1 cup

Mung beans are small green beans that can be eaten with butter or spices as sprouts or ground into flour (cooking time 25 to 40 minutes). Like all legumes they are very nutritious and have exceptionally low GI values. Indian green gram dahl is a favorite ethnic dish based on mashed, cooked mung beans. They are a good source of dietary fiber, iron, and protein and also contain vitamin C.

Navy Beans, Cooked

■

GI Value	38
Glycemic Load	12

Carbohydrate	31 g
Fat	1 g
Fiber	12 g

Serving size • 1 cup

Navy beans are used for making baked beans and are an excellent source of fiber, protein, iron, potassium, and zinc. If you make your own baked beans, they'll have a lower GI value than the canned version. Legumes of all sorts, including navy beans, are renowned for producing flatulence (gas). The components responsible are indigestible sugars called raffinose, stachyose, and verbascose. They reach the large bowel intact where they are fermented by the resident microflora. Believe it or not, this is good for colon health, increasing the proportion of good *Bifidobacteria* and reducing any potential pathogens. The commercial product Beano helps to break down intestinal gas.

Nutella ®

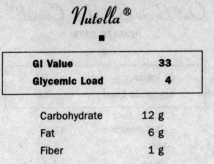

GI Value	33
Glycemic Load	4

Carbohydrate	12 g
Fat	6 g
Fiber	1 g

Serving size • 1 tablespoon

*N*utella® is a sweetened chocolate spread based on hazelnuts that's a favorite even among non-chocoholics. Its fat content is high but the fats are mainly mono- and polyunsaturated, so it can be a healthy addition to the balanced diet of any active person. Nutella®'s low GI value results from its rich mixture of fat and sugars—high concentrations of both slow down stomach emptying.

Oat Bran Breakfast Cereal™
(QUAKER OATS)

■

GI Value	50
Glycemic Load	10

Carbohydrate	19 g
Fat	1 g
Fiber	4 g

Serving size • ¾ cup

Quaker Oats Oat Bran Breakfast Cereal™ is just like the hot bran cereal except that it contains dry flakes of natural oat bran and whole-grain wheat. The oat bran contains soluble fiber, which is believed to lower cholesterol and reduce the risk of heart disease when included as part of a high-fiber, low-fat diet. Add fresh or natural canned fruit and skim or 1% milk and you'll start your day with an energy-packed and nutritionally dense breakfast.

Oat Bran, Raw
(QUAKER OATS)

■

GI Value	**55**
Glycemic Load	**3**

Carbohydrate	6 g
Fat	1 g
Fiber	2 g

Serving size • 1 tablespoon

*U*nprocessed oat bran is available in the cereal section of supermarkets or in health food stores. Its carbohydrate content is lower than that of oats and it is higher in fiber, particularly soluble fiber, which is responsible for its low GI value. When mixed with water, oat bran forms a jellylike mixture that increases the viscosity (or movement) of the solution in the small intestine. This slows down the movement of enzymes and food, resulting in slower digestion. A soft, bland product, oat bran is a useful addition to breakfast cereals and as a partial substitution for flour in baked goods to help lower the food's GI value.

Oatmeal Cookies

■

GI Value	**54**
Glycemic Load	**9**

Carbohydrate	17 g
Fat	5 g
Fiber	1 g

Serving size • One 1-oz cookie

*Th*e use of rolled oats, along with some sugar and added fat, is probably why oatmeal cookies have a low GI value. Nutritionists explain that there is, in fact, a place for cookies in a balanced meal plan as long as the portion is small. Oatmeal cookies make an excellent low-GI choice to satisfy that sweet tooth after a balanced meal or as a healthy snack.

Oatmeal, Old-Fashioned

■

GI Value	51
Glycemic Load	11

Carbohydrate	21 g
Fat	2 g
Fiber	4 g

Serving size • 1 cup cooked

Old-fashioned cooked oats are a good source of viscous soluble fiber, B vitamins, vitamin E, iron, and zinc. Rolled oats are hulled, steamed, and flattened, which makes oatmeal a 100% whole-grain cereal. The additional flaking of rolled oats to produce quick-cooking oats increases the rate of digestion, which results in a higher GI value. This is why old-fashioned oats are preferred over quick or instant. Supplementing a low-fat diet with rolled oats can help lower cholesterol. Cooking the oats in milk (preferably skim or 1%) not only produces a creamy cooked cereal but also supplies you with 30 mg of calcium. Add fresh or unsweetened canned fruit for a high-energy breakfast.

Orange Marmalade

■

GI Value	**48**
Glycemic Load	**9**

Carbohydrate	20 g
Fat	0 g
Fiber	0 g

Serving size • 1½ tablespoons

*M*armalade is a fruit jelly that contains unpeeled pieces of fruit—usually citrus, but it may also contain peaches, pineapples, or cranberries. To prepare orange marmalade, the fruit is sliced and cooked in water for some time before the sugar is added. It has cooked enough when it reaches a jelled stage. This delicious fruit condiment derives its low GI value from its two constituent parts: oranges (GI = 48) and sugar (GI = 61). Orange marmalade is a sweet-tasting condiment that anyone can include in their diet.

Oranges, Navel

■

GI Value	48
Glycemic Load	5

Carbohydrate	11 g
Fat	0 g
Fiber	3 g

Serving size • 1 small (4 oz)

*O*ranges are a major source of vitamin C: One orange can provide around 60 mg of vitamin C! Much of an orange's sugar content is sucrose, a "double" sugar made up of glucose and fructose. When it's digested, only the glucose molecule impacts blood-sugar levels. This and the high acid content account for the orange's low GI value.

Pasta

MOST PASTA IS made from semolina (cracked wheat), which is milled from very hard wheat with a high protein content. Durum wheat is a hard, high-protein wheat that is considered the best for making pasta. A stiff dough is made by mixing the semolina with water, which is forced through a die and dried. There is minimal mechanical disruption of the starch granule during this process and strong protein-starch interactions inhibit starch gelatinization. The dense consistency also makes the pasta resistant to disruption in the small intestine and contributes to its ultimately low GI value—even pasta made from fine flour instead of semolina has a relatively low GI value. There is some evidence that thicker pasta has a lower GI value than thin types for this reason. The addition of egg to fresh pasta lowers the glycemic index value by increasing the protein content. Higher protein levels inhibit stomach emptying.

With all the current controversy over high vs. low carb intake, the focus centers on the amount of carbs you consume. It's how quickly the carbs you eat reach your bloodstream that determines your energy level and appetite.

Any pasta, cooked al dente, will not cause blood-sugar spikes when you eat moderate portions. One cup of cooked pasta—which can turn into three cups on your plate by mixing in primavera vegetables, for example—can fit into any adult's daily diet.

Pastina

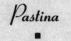

■

GI Value	**38**
Glycemic Load	**18**

Carbohydrate	48 g
Fat	<1 g
Fiber	2 g

Serving size • 1 cup cooked

Small pasta or "pastina" comes in many shapes: stars, *orzo, acini di pepe,* and many more. But just like the larger shaped pasta (including spaghetti, macaroni, ziti, and elbows), they are all made from durum wheat semolina, which is a low-GI carbohydrate. Pastinas are used in vegetable, chicken, and beef broths to provide some thickeners and added calories to the soup. Children particularly love the shapes of these smaller pastas.

Peaches, Canned in Natural Juice

■

GI Value	**38**
Glycemic Load	**4**

Carbohydrate	11 g
Fat	0 g
Fiber	2 g

Serving size • ½ cup

Peaches canned in natural juice have a low glycemic index value. This is probably attributable to a high fructose content and high osmolality (osmotic pressure) that slows stomach emptying. Single-serving cans with flip-open tabs make peaches easy to eat away from home.

Peaches, Fresh

■

GI Value	**42**
Glycemic Load	**5**

Carbohydrate	11 g
Fat	0 g
Fiber	2 g

Serving size • 1 medium

*M*uch of the sugar in peaches is sucrose, which is identical to normal table sugar. It is a "double" sugar made up of glucose and fructose. When digested, only the glucose molecule affects blood-sugar levels. This fact, along with the soluble fiber content and natural acidity, accounts for peaches' low GI value. A peach is a good source of vitamins A and C, niacin, and potassium. Since peaches are often coated with a thin layer of wax to prolong shelf life, wash them well before eating or peel them and poach them in white wine.

Peanut Butter
∎

GI Value	**14**
Glycemic Load	**7**

Carbohydrate	5 g
Fat	16 g
Fiber	2 g

Serving size • 2 tablespoons

Ground peanuts result in the delicious treat we know as peanut butter. When left to settle, the oil in the peanuts separates from the peanut mash, or paste. The healthiest type of peanut butter has no added sugar, salt, or heart-unhealthy emulsifiers (used to prevent oil separation). Natural peanut butter has a very low GI value because of its negligible carbohydrate content, which is the same type found in peas and beans, since peanuts are technically legumes. Peanut butter is an excellent source of niacin and a good source of magnesium. A recent study from the Harvard University School of Public Health found that increased nut consumption, including natural peanut butter, may improve the body's ability to balance glucose and insulin, and also lower cholesterol. The healthiest way to include more peanut butter into your diet is to eat it regularly *in place of* refined grain products or high-fat protein foods and processed meats. For example, it's healthier to eat one or two tablespoons of peanut butter on whole-grain bread instead of a bowl of highly processed breakfast cereal or to eat a peanut butter and jelly sandwich instead of a hamburger, grilled cheese, or egg-salad sandwich.

Peanuts

■

GI Value	14
Glycemic Load	1

Carbohydrate	6 g
Fat	25 g
Fiber	4 g

Serving size • 1.75-oz package

A low-carbohydrate but high-fat, high-protein food (50 percent fat and 25 percent protein), peanuts grow under the ground (they are also known as groundnuts). They are an excellent source of vitamins E and B. They're so low in carbohydrate that their glycemic index value doesn't really count, although their high fat content does. Because peanuts are such a convenient and tasty finger food, it's easy to eat too many of them. All processed peanuts are quality controlled for the presence of fungus, because fungus produces a toxin called aflatoxin, one of the most carcinogenic substances known. Because peanuts in the shell *aren't* screened, be sure never to eat a moldy peanut. A word to the wise: Choose dry-roasted nuts and avoid the salt.

Pears, Canned in Natural Juice
■

GI Value	49
Glycemic Load	5

Carbohydrate	11 g
Fat	0 g
Fiber	2 g

Serving size • ½ cup

The GI value of a canned pear is only slightly higher than that of the fresh fruit. This is because fructose, the low-GI natural sugar found in fruit, remains in high concentration in the pears even when they are canned. Pears are rich in fiber, potassium, and copper. Dehydrated or dried pears, now more commonly found in the produce departments of supermarkets and in health food stores, contain an even more concentrated supply of valuable vitamins and minerals.

Pears, Fresh

■

GI Value	**38**
Glycemic Load	**4**

Carbohydrate	11 g
Fat	0 g
Fiber	2 g

Serving size • ½ medium

*P*ears have a high amount of fructose, a sugar with a minimal effect on blood-sugar levels. Pears are at their peak during autumn. They ripen quickly and should be eaten before they get too soft. They are a nice accompaniment to cheese and walnuts, or poached or baked in a syrup or red wine; try adding a pinch of cardamom for an exquisite combination of flavors.

Peas, Green, Frozen

■

GI Value	**48**
Glycemic Load	**3**

Carbohydrate	7 g
Fat	<1 g
Fiber	4 g

Serving size • ½ cup cooked

*P*eas are properly classified as legumes. They are high in fiber and also higher in protein than most other vegetables. More amylose, lower degrees of starch gelatinization, and protein-starch interactions may contribute to their lower glycemic index value. While most of the carbohydrate is starch, they also contain sucrose, which gives them a sweet flavor.

Pinto Beans, Canned

∎

GI Value	**45**
Glycemic Load	**10**

Carbohydrate	22 g
Fat	1 g
Fiber	7 g

Serving size • ⅔ cup

The canning process slightly raises the GI value of pinto beans by permitting greater swelling or gelatinization of the starch molecules, which increases the rate of digestion and absorption. Canned pinto beans remain, however, a great low-GI food choice. These versatile beans are used as vegetable side dishes, or are added to soups, salads, and stews. Their flavor blends particularly well with tomatoes, thyme, oregano, rosemary, mint marjoram, mustard, nutmeg, and cardamom.

Plums, Fresh

■

GI Value	39
Glycemic Load	5

Carbohydrate	12 g
Fat	0 g
Fiber	1 g

Serving size • 1 large

The combination of organic acids and a high concentration of sugars in plums slows down the rate of stomach emptying, which reduces your body's glycemic response to this fruit. Plums also contain viscous fiber, which reduces the rate of digestion in the small intestine. They make a light, tasty snack—as do prunes, the dried version of this fruit.

Potatoes—Which to Choose

BOILED, MASHED, BAKED, grilled, or fried—everyone loves potatoes in one form or another. Unfortunately, just about any potato found in your grocery store has a high GI value (greater than 78). The only potatoes with a lower GI value are the tiny, new, canned variety (GI = 65). The lower glycemic index value of new potatoes may be due to differences in the structure of the starch. As potatoes age, the degree of branching of their amylopectin starch increases significantly, becoming more readily gelatinized and digested, thus producing a higher GI value. New potatoes are also smaller than mature potatoes and a correlation has been found between the size of the potato and its glycemic index value—the smaller the potato, the lower the GI value.

So we suggest that you eat small, new potatoes if you love spuds, and focus on eating other low-GI foods that day. Vary your diet with other sources of carbohydrate—rice, pasta, and legumes. And remember, potatoes are fat free, nutritious, and very satisfying, and not everything has to have a low GI value—so enjoy them!

Although they're not potatoes at all, some people eat sweet potatoes and yams in place of their white potatoes. (See "Sweet Potato" on page 128 and "Yam" on page 133 for more information about these tubers.)

Pound Cake

◾

GI Value	**54**
Glycemic Load	**15**

Carbohydrate	28 g
Fat	9 g
Fiber	0 g

Serving size • ⅟₁₆ loaf

The name "pound cake" comes from the traditional recipe, which includes equal weights (one pound) of each of its key ingredients: flour, butter, and sugar. Today's bakers have modified the traditional recipe, but pound cake retains its dense consistency and rich, buttery flavor. The relatively high proportion of sugar decreases the amount of starch gelatinization (swelling), which produces a more gradual release of glucose into the blood after the cake is digested. The presence of a considerable amount of fat (from butter and/or margarine) also slows the movement of glucose molecules from the intestine into the blood. To increase the nutrient density of this low-GI dessert, add sliced fresh fruit and low-fat yogurt.

Prunes, Dried

■

GI Value	**29**
Glycemic Load	**10**

Carbohydrate	33 g
Fat	0 g
Fiber	4 g

Serving size • 7

There are just a few plum varieties that dry well without requiring the removal of their stone. Whether dried in the sun or industrially, these dried plums are known as prunes. It's the high sugar content, the naturally occurring acids, and the presence of insoluble fibers that make prunes a low-GI food. Prunes offer many nutritional benefits: They're rich in vitamin A, several B vitamins, vitamin C, and abundant minerals, including potassium, iron, magnesium, and calcium. They are commonly added to lamb, pork, chicken, and game dishes. They're easy to carry along for a snack and, when cooked or eaten before bedtime, dried prunes have a strong laxative effect.

Pudding, Cook and Serve, Sugar Free

■

GI Value	**43**
Glycemic Load	**6**

Carbohydrate	13 g
Fat	0 g
Fiber	0 g

Serving size • ½ cup

When cooked with skim or 1% milk, sugar-free pudding in any flavor is a sweet-tasting, nutritious, low-GI dessert that provides 150 mg of calcium. Because the primary carbohydrate source (cornstarch) has not been modified to reduce the cooking time, the chemical breakdown into glucose is slower, which is why cooked puddings have lower GI values than instant varieties. If you're looking for a sweet, low-GI dessert idea, cooked sugar-free puddings might be the answer.

Ravioli, Meat-Filled

■

GI Value	**39**
Glycemic Load	**15**

Carbohydrate	38 g
Fat	13 g
Fiber	4 g

Serving size • 1 cup cooked

*Y*ou can buy ravioli fresh, frozen, or vacuum packed, with any number of delicious fillings. A homemade tomato and basil sauce with a sprinkle of Parmesan cheese is a classic ravioli dish. What makes it even better is that by adding a large salad and fruit dessert, you will have assembled a low-GI meal in less than twenty minutes! Other ravioli fillings include cheese, spinach, tofu, butternut squash, pumpkin, and mushrooms.

Salad Vegetables

SALAD VEGETABLES SUCH as lettuce, tomatoes, cucumber, radishes, mushrooms, peppers, and onions have so little carbohydrate that it's impossible to test their glycemic index value (50 g carbohydrate portions would be more than two pounds, worth!). Even in generous serving sizes, salad vegetables have no effect on blood-glucose levels and should be regarded as "free" foods that are full of healthy nutrients.

Rice Bran

■

GI Value	**19**
Glycemic Load	**1**

Carbohydrate	2 g
Fat	2 g
Fiber	2 g

Serving size • 1 tablespoon

Rice bran is a good source of thiamin, riboflavin, and niacin and has a sweet malty flavor. Rice bran is actually the outer bran layer that is scraped from brown rice in the milling of white rice, and it contains the fibrous seed coat and a small part of the germ. It is rich in fiber (25 percent by weight) and oil (20 percent by weight) and has an extremely low GI value. Rice bran is available in the cereal section of supermarkets or in health food stores. Sprinkle it on breakfast cereal or add to baked goods or meatloaf for extra fiber and nutrients.

Rice, Brown

■

GI Value	**50**
Glycemic Load	**16**

Carbohydrate	33 g
Fat	0 g
Fiber	4 g

Serving size • 1 cup cooked

Brown rice is the whole rice grain with just the inedible outer shell removed. Brown rice is the most nutritious form of rice, because it contains several B vitamins and minerals, dietary fiber, and protein. Its compact structure and fibrous nature make it an excellent low-GI food choice, and also make it chewier than regular white rice. Like all low-GI foods, this rice will curtail your hunger for hours after you eat it—in other words, a little goes a long way!

Rice, Converted Long Grain, Parboiled

(UNCLE BEN'S™)

◾

GI Value	**38**
Glycemic Load	**14**

Carbohydrate	36 g
Fat	<1 g
Fiber	1 g

Serving size • ⅔ cup cooked

Parboiled or converted long-grain white rice is soaked, then steamed, before being milled. This process transfers the B vitamins and minerals that are contained in the germ and outer layers to the interior of the grain. Converted or parboiled rice is second only to brown rice in its nutritional quality. In addition, its high amylose starch content gives it its low GI value. You can use converted rice in any of the same ways (and in the same dishes) you would other types of rice.

Rice, Long Grain and Wild
(UNCLE BEN'S™)

■

GI Value	**54**
Glycemic Load	**20**

Carbohydrate	37 g
Fat	0 g
Fiber	1 g

Serving size • ⅔ cup cooked

Long-grain rice is light and delicate. One bonus for cooks is that the grains also remain separate when they're cooked. No more clumps! Like the other low-GI rices, the compact structure and high amylose starch content contribute to long-grain rice's slow digestion rate. Wild rice is actually not rice at all, but rather a type of grass. Delicious as a side dish, many people also add long-grain white rice to casseroles and use them to make fried rice cakes and cold rice salads, as well. You can find this common mix of grains at most supermarkets.

Semolina

■

GI Value	**55**
Glycemic Load	**9**

Carbohydrate	17 g
Fat	0 g
Fiber	0 g

Serving size • 1 cup cooked

Semolina is the coarsely milled inner part of the wheat grain called the endosperm. It is granular in appearance. The large particle size of semolina flour (compared with fine wheat flour) limits the swelling of its starch particles when it's cooked, which results in slower digestion rates and slower release of sugar into the bloodstream.

You'll find durum wheat semolina in most supermarkets. You can use it to make homemade pasta or to cook and eat as a hot cereal. As instant flour, you can use semolina to thicken sauces and gravies.

Social Tea Biscuits ™
(NABISCO)

■

GI Value	**55**
Glycemic Load	**10**

Carbohydrate	19 g
Fat	4 g
Fiber	1 g

Serving size • 6 cookies

*S*ocial Tea Biscuits™ are thin, sweet cookies. What makes this a low-GI snack? Cookie dough has a low water-to-flour ratio and a high sugar content, which results in lower levels of starch gelatinization than in most bread dough. All things considered, cookies, whether high or low in sugar, are packed with calories and taste great, so it's easy to overeat them. Eat these in moderation.

Soybeans

∎

GI Value	**14**
Glycemic Load	**1**

Carbohydrate	2 g
Fat	6 g
Fiber	5 g

Serving size • ½ cup

Soybeans contain substantial amounts of fiber, iron, zinc, and vitamin B and are an excellent source of protein. They are also higher in fat than other legumes, but the majority of this fat is polyunsaturated. They are quite low in carbohydrate. Soybeans also contain phytoestrogens (a type of plant estrogen similar in structure to the female hormone estrogen, but with a much weaker action). Many studies associate soybeans with beneficial effects—improvements in blood-cholesterol levels, alleviation of some menopausal symptoms, lower risk of breast cancer. (You would need to eat two to three servings of soy a day to achieve these benefits.)

You can buy soybeans dried (you'll need to soak and then boil them for about two hours), canned, or roasted. You can also enjoy them as soybean curd (tofu), soybean flour, tempeh, miso, or textured vegetable protein (TVP), which you can find in some veggie burgers. All of these forms of soybeans have little carbohydrate and therefore minimal effects on blood-sugar levels. Flavored soy milks are becoming increasingly popular, too; see the "Vitasoy" entry on page 119.

Soy Milk
(VITASOY®)

GI Value	**31**
Glycemic Load	**3**

Carbohydrate	10 g
Fat	5 g
Fiber	1 g

Serving size • 1 cup (8 oz)

Soy milk is a completely dairy- and lactose-free milk. Whole soybeans—which are often organically grown— are mixed with filtered water and flavorings to produce a milklike product. Once enjoyed only by vegetarians, soy milk has become increasingly popular, possibly because it tastes good and is recognized to be rich in isoflavones, nutrients that are known to have health benefits. (See the "Soybeans" entry on page 118 for more information about these benefits.)

Spaghetti with Meat Sauce
•

GI Value	**52**
Glycemic Load	**25**

Carbohydrate	48 g
Fat	5 g
Fiber	3 g

Serving size • 1 cup cooked

Spaghetti is probably the best known and most widely consumed of all the forms of pasta made from durum wheat or semolina flour. Its sturdy texture, which comes from the high gluten content of the durum wheat, allows for a slow release of glucose molecules as it is broken down. A low-fat meat sauce, made from lean cuts of beef, pork, or veal, tomatoes, carrots, onions, celery, and fresh herbs, placed on top of cooked spaghetti, is a popular, nutrient-dense entrée. Because of its versatility, spaghetti is the perfect accompaniment to meat-, chicken-, or fish-based, vegetable-based, or oil-based sauces—all of which fit into a healthy, balanced diet.

Spaghetti, Durum Wheat

■

GI Value	**42**
Glycemic Load	**20**

Carbohydrate	47 g
Fat	1 g
Fiber	3 g

Serving size • 1 cup cooked

Spaghetti is probably the most popular form of pasta. Like all pasta, spaghetti has a low GI value because the dough is made from high-protein semolina (large particles of wheat) and because of its dense food matrix, which resists disruption in the small intestine. Both fresh and dried spaghetti are low-GI foods. Spaghetti's versatility is endless: It blends beautifully with cooked and raw vegetables; any mixture of herbs and spices; meats, poultry, fish, and shellfish; and sauces containing olive oil, margarine, butter, or light cream; and even nuts such as walnuts, pine nuts, and sunflower seeds. Canned spaghetti, which is usually made from flour rather than semolina—and is very well cooked—has a higher GI value.

Spaghetti, Whole Wheat

■

GI Value	32
Glycemic Load	14

Carbohydrate	44 g
Fat	<1 g
Fiber	5 g

Serving size • 1¼ cups cooked

All the low-GI virtues of regular enriched spaghetti apply to whole-wheat spaghetti and for the same reasons. These two types of pasta can be interchanged in any recipe; you can enjoy this spaghetti with all the same sauces and accompaniments as you would white. Just keep in mind that you'll be getting more than double the amount of dietary fiber when you eat whole wheat spaghetti instead of white spaghetti made from durum wheat.

Split Peas, Dried

■

GI Value	32
Glycemic Load	6

Carbohydrate	19 g
Fat	<1 g
Fiber	12 g

Serving size • ¾ cup cooked

All 1,000-plus varieties of peas technically belong to the legume plant family. Dried peas are a storehouse of nutrition and because their calories are slowly digested (which makes them a low-GI food), a little goes a long way. They take about one hour to cook after soaking and tend to disintegrate if they're overcooked. Their low GI value is due to a combination of factors: Higher amylose content; physical entrapment of starch inside the cell wall of the seed; lower levels of starch gelatinization during cooking; and higher levels of substances that inhibit enzymes (such as tannins).

Sponge Cake

■

GI Value	**46**
Glycemic Load	**17**

Carbohydrate	36 g
Fat	3 g
Fiber	0 g

Serving size • ¹⁄₁₂ of 10-inch cake

Sponge cake is similar to angel food cake, but with egg yolks added. The low glycemic index value of sponge cake results because the starch molecules don't swell very much in this recipe and, therefore, break down slowly. If this cake is a real favorite, try replacing some of the yolks with an egg substitute.

Strawberries, Fresh

▪

GI Value	**40**
Glycemic Load	**1**

Carbohydrate	3 g
Fat	0 g
Fiber	3 g

Serving size • ¾ cup sliced

At only 3 percent carbohydrate and 92 percent water, the average pint of strawberries provides less than two teaspoons of natural sugars. These berries are rich in vitamin C, potassium, folic acid, and fiber.

About half the carbohydrate in strawberries comes from glucose and half from fructose—there is no sucrose. The low glycemic index value of strawberries might be due to both their soluble fiber content and relative acidity.

The average one-cup serving has very little impact on blood-glucose levels, which makes them a fruit to enjoy when they're in season. Try fresh strawberries cut into quarters and macerated with balsamic vinegar and sugar. A fresh strawberry puree makes a great sauce over vanilla ice cream. Just don't eat too many strawberries in a single day: they can have diuretic and laxative effects if you eat too many of them.

Strawberry Jam

■

GI Value	**51**
Glycemic Load	**10**

Carbohydrate	20 g
Fat	0 g
Fiber	0 g

Serving size • 1½ tablespoons

*M*aking jam is an effective way to preserve the fresh, delicate flavors of some fruits. Small in size, strawberries make a perfect choice to mash, chop, or dice for making jam. The high sugar content and the low GI value of the strawberries (GI = 40) make strawberry jam an excellent fruit-based complement to any balanced diet.

Sushi

■

GI Value	52
Glycemic Load	19

Carbohydrate	37 g
Fat	2 g
Fiber	2 g

Serving size • 5 pieces

Japanese sushi is bite-sized pieces of raw or smoked fish, chicken, tofu, or pickled, raw, or cooked vegetables wrapped in seaweed with rice that has been seasoned with vinegar, salt, and sugar.

Even though the rice used to make sushi is short grain and somewhat sticky, sushi still has a low GI value, possibly because of the presence of vinegar (acidity puts the brakes on stomach emptying) and the viscous fiber in the dried seaweed. Sushi made with salmon and tuna contributes to higher intakes of beneficial very long-chain polyunsaturated fats such as DHA and EPA.

Sweet Potato

■

GI Value	**48**
Glycemic Load	**16**

Carbohydrate	34 g
Fat	<1 g
Fiber	4 g

Serving size • 1 small (5 oz)

The orange-colored sweet potato is an excellent source of beta-carotene, the plant precursor of vitamin A. Sweet potato is also a good source of vitamin C and fiber. The sweet flavor comes from naturally present sucrose. Its low GI value is associated with increased amounts of amylose.

Sweet potatoes belong to a different plant family than regular white potatoes—would you believe, the morning glory family? Prepare and cook them as you would ordinary potatoes—steam, boil, mash, bake, grill, or fry them. They're also tasty additions to casseroles, stir-fries, and soups.

Tomato Juice, No Sugar Added
■

GI Value	38
Glycemic Load	4

Carbohydrate	9 g
Fat	0 g
Fiber	1 g

Serving size • 1 cup (8 oz)

Tomato juice is a fantastic low-GI, low-calorie replacement for carbonated beverages. For fewer than 40 calories, an 8-ounce glass of thirst-quenching tomato juice provides vitamins A and C, potassium, and folic acid. The low GI value of this healthy beverage is due to its acidity and the presence of sucrose, although the amounts of each depend on the type of tomatoes used. On the rocks or straight from the can, you can feel good about drinking tomato juice (with no sugar and minimal sodium added) frequently.

Tomato Soup, Canned

■

GI Value	38
Glycemic Load	6

Carbohydrate	17 g
Fat	4 g
Fiber	4 g

Serving size • 1 cup (8 oz)

Canned tomato soups tend to contain large amounts of sodium, so look for salt-reduced varieties when purchasing your next can. Besides making an easy meal with some low-GI toast and a hearty salad, tomato soup can be used undiluted in many casserole recipes. Its low GI value is related to its acidity and the bulk of its carbohydrate being sucrose.

Tortellini, Cheese, Frozen

■

GI Value	50
Glycemic Load	10

Carbohydrate	21 g
Fat	15 g
Fiber	5 g

Serving size • 6-oz entrée

Tortellini is a small, crescent-shaped filled pasta with an unlimited range of fillings. Some popular fillings include spinach and ricotta, chicken, veal, ham, mushrooms, and cheese. Tortellini is usually bought fresh, frozen, or vacuum packed. It is boiled, then served with a sauce or melted butter, fresh herbs, and grated cheese. The nutrient content will vary depending on the type of filling. Like all pasta, tortellini has a low GI value.

Vegetables

YOU CAN EAT most vegetables without thinking about their glycemic index value. You should eat at least four servings of different vegetables daily. Most veggies are so low in carbohydrate that they have no measurable effect on blood-glucose levels, though they still provide valuable amounts of vitamins and minerals. Because of their high fiber content, veggies also help us feel full longer.

Higher-carbohydrate vegetables include potato, sweet potato, and corn. Among these, corn and sweet potato are the lower-GI choices. Pumpkin, carrots, peas, and beets contain some carbohydrate, but a normal serving contains so little that it doesn't raise blood-glucose levels significantly. So eat, enjoy, and feel good about improving your health and your diet!

Yam

▪

GI Value	37
Glycemic Load	13

Carbohydrate	36 g
Fat	<1 g
Fiber	6 g

Serving size • 1 small (5 oz)

The edible roots of climbing plants, yams are a good source of vitamin C and potassium. They are similar to sweet potato and can be prepared in similar ways—boiled, baked, grilled, or stir-fried. In fact, you can use yams in place of sweet or white potatoes in most recipes. The low GI value is related to a higher proportion of amylose in the starch content.

What's the Difference between a Sweet Potato and a Yam?

BOTH VEGETABLES ARE tubers, though they come from different families. The most popular type of sweet potato (there are more than 400 varieties) has a smooth reddish-orange skin and orange flesh. The yam, which can grow to a weight of 45 pounds, has a thick, brownish skin and creamy inner flesh. Yams have a more earthy and less sweet flavor than the sweet potato. Both are high-fiber, nutrient-dense, low-GI foods.

Yogurt, Low-fat, with Fruit and Artificial Sweetener

■

GI Value	**14**
Glycemic Load	**2**

Carbohydrate	13 g
Fat	2 g
Fiber	0 g

Serving size • 6-oz container

All varieties of yogurt have low glycemic index values. When sweetened artificially, flavored yogurt has an even lower GI value and contains fewer calories than naturally sweetened yogurt. Low-fat yogurt provides the most calcium for the fewest calories. When yogurt is made, the bacterial cultures that are added to the milk break down some of the sugar lactose into the lactic acid, which denatures the protein and forms a soft curd. The acidity and high protein content slow down stomach emptying, contributing to its low GI value. The remaining lactose itself has a low GI value, so it doesn't greatly affect yogurt's final GI value. Lactose-intolerant people can eat yogurt without experiencing abdominal distress.

◄ 6 ►

A TO Z GI VALUES

THE TABLE IN this section will help you find a food's glycemic index value quickly and easily, because we've listed the foods alphabetically.

The list provides not only the food's glycemic index value but also its glycemic load (GL = (carbohydrate content × GI) ÷ 100). We calculate the glycemic load using a nominal, or standardized, serving size as well as the carbohydrate content of that serving—both of which we've also listed. That way, you can choose foods with either a low GI value or a low glycemic load. If your favorite food is both high GI and high GL, you can either cut down the serving size or dilute the GL by combining it with very low-GI foods, such as rice and lentils.

For the first time, we've also included foods that have very little carbohydrate; their GI value is zero, indicated by [0]. Many vegetables, such as avocados and broccoli, and protein foods such as chicken, cheese, and tuna, fall

into the low- or no-carbohydrate category. Most alcoholic beverages are also low in carbohydrate.

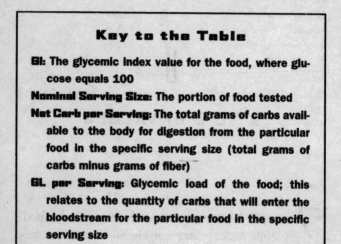

Key to the Table

GI: The glycemic index value for the food, where glucose equals 100

Nominal Serving Size: The portion of food tested

Net Carb per Serving: The total grams of carbs available to the body for digestion from the particular
food in the specific serving size (total grams of
carbs minus grams of fiber)

GL per Serving: Glycemic load of the food; this
relates to the quantity of carbs that will enter the
bloodstream for the particular food in the specific
serving size

FOOD	GI Value	Nominal Serving Size	Net Carb per Serving	GL per Serving
A				
All-Bran®, breakfast cereal	30	½ cup	15	4
Almonds	[0]	1.75 oz	0	0
Angel food cake, 1 slice	67	1/12 cake	29	19
Apple, dried	29	9 rings	34	10
Apple, fresh, medium	38	4 oz	15	6
Apple juice, pure, unsweetened, reconstituted	40	8 oz	29	12
Apple muffin, small	44	3.5 oz	41	18
Apricots, canned in light syrup	64	4 halves	19	12
Apricots, dried	30	17 halves	27	8
Apricots, fresh, 3 medium	57	4 oz	9	5
Arborio, risotto rice, cooked	69	¾ cup	53	36
Artichokes (Jerusalem)	[0]	½ cup	0	0
Avocado	[0]	¼	0	0
B				
Bagel, white	72	½	35	25
Baked beans	38	⅔ cup	31	12
Baked beans, canned in tomato sauce	48	⅔ cup	15	7
Banana cake, 1 slice	47	⅛ cake	38	18
Banana, fresh, medium	52	4 oz	24	12
Barley, pearled, cooked	25	1 cup	42	11
Basmati rice, white, cooked	58	1 cup	38	22
Beef	[0]	4 oz	0	0
Beer	[0]	8 oz	10	0
Beets, canned	64	½ cup	7	5
Bengal gram dhal, chickpea	11	5 oz	36	4
Black bean soup	64	1 cup	27	17
Black beans, cooked	30	⅘ cup	23	7
Black-eyed peas, canned	42	⅔ cup	17	7

[0] indicates that the food has so little carbohydrate that the GI value cannot be tested. The GL, therefore, is 0.

FOOD	GI Value	Nominal Serving Size	Net Carb per Serving	GL per Serving
Blueberry muffin, small	59	3.5 oz	47	28
Bok choy, raw	[0]	1 cup	0	0
Bran Flakes™, breakfast cereal	74	½ cup	18	13
Bran muffin, small	60	3.5 oz	41	25
Brandy	[0]	1 oz	0	0
Brazil nuts	[0]	1.75 oz	0	0
Breton wheat crackers	67	6 crackers	14	10
Broad beans	79	½ cup	11	9
Broccoli, raw	[0]	1 cup	0	0
Broken rice, white, cooked	86	1 cup	43	37
Brown rice, cooked	50	1 cup	33	16
Buckwheat	54	¾ cup	30	16
Bulgur, cooked 20 min	48	¾ cup	26	12
Bun, hamburger	61	1.5 oz	22	13
Butter beans, canned	31	⅔ cup	20	6

C

FOOD	GI Value	Nominal Serving Size	Net Carb per Serving	GL per Serving
Cabbage, raw	[0]	1 cup	0	0
Cactus Nectar, Organic Agave, light, 90% fructose (Western Commerce)	11	1 Tbsp	8	1
Cactus Nectar, Organic Agave, light, 97% fructose (Western Commerce)	10	1 Tbsp	8	1
Cantaloupe, fresh	85	4 oz	6	4
Cappellini pasta, cooked	45	1½ cups	45	20
Carrot juice, fresh	43	8 oz	23	10
Carrots, peeled, cooked	49	½ cup	5	2
Carrots, raw	47	1 medium	6	3
Cashew nuts, salted	22	1.75 oz	13	3
Cauliflower, raw	[0]	¾ cup	0	0
Celery, raw	[0]	2 stalks	0	0
Cheese	[0]	4 oz	0	0

[0] indicates that the food has so little carbohydrate that the GI value cannot be tested. The GL, therefore, is 0.

FOOD	GI Value	Nominal Serving Size	Net Carb per Serving	GL per Serving
Cherries, fresh	22	18	12	3
Chicken nuggets, frozen	46	4 oz	16	7
Chickpeas, canned	42	⅔ cup	22	9
Chickpeas, dried, cooked	28	⅔ cup	30	8
Chocolate cake made from mix with chocolate frosting	38	4 oz	52	20
Chocolate milk, low-fat	34	8 oz	26	9
Chocolate mousse, 2% fat	31	½ cup	22	7
Chocolate powder, dissolved in water	55	8 oz	16	9
Chocolate pudding, made from powder and whole milk	47	½ cup	24	11
Choice DM™, nutritional support product, vanilla (Mead Johnson)	23	8 oz	24	6
Clif® bar (cookies & cream)	101	2.4 oz	34	34
Coca Cola®, soft drink	53	8 oz	26	14
Cocoa Puffs™, breakfast cereal	77	1 cup	26	20
Complete™, breakfast cereal	48	1 cup	21	10
Condensed milk, sweetened	61	2½ Tbsps	27	17
Converted rice, long-grain, cooked 20-30 min, Uncle Ben's®	50	1 cup	36	18
Converted rice, white, cooked 20-30 min, Uncle Ben's®	38	1 cup	36	14
Corn Flakes™, breakfast cereal	92	1 cup	26	24
Corn Flakes™, Honey Crunch, breakfast cereal	72	¾ cup	25	18
Corn pasta, gluten-free	78	1¼ cups	42	32
Corn Pops™, breakfast cereal	80	1 cup	26	21
Corn Thins, puffed corn cakes, gluten-free	87	1 oz	20	18
Corn, sweet, cooked	60	½ cup	18	11
Cornmeal, cooked 2 min	68	1 cup	13	9
Couscous, cooked 5 min	65	¾ cup	35	23

[0] indicates that the food has so little carbohydrate that the GI value cannot be tested. The GL, therefore, is 0.

FOOD	GI Value	Nominal Serving Size	Net Carb per Serving	GL per Serving
Cranberry juice cocktail	52	8 oz	31	16
Crispix™, breakfast cereal	87	1 cup	25	22
Croissant, medium	67	2 oz	26	17
Cucumber, raw	[0]	¾ cup	0	0
Cupcake, strawberry-iced, small	73	1.5 oz	26	19
Custard apple, raw, flesh only	54	4 oz	19	10
Custard, homemade	43	½ cup	26	11
Custard, prepared from powder with whole milk, instant	35	½ cup	26	9

D

FOOD	GI Value	Nominal Serving Size	Net Carb per Serving	GL per Serving
Dates, dried	50	7	40	20
Desiree potato, peeled, cooked	101	5 oz	17	17
Doughnut, cake type	76	1.75 oz	23	17

E

FOOD	GI Value	Nominal Serving Size	Net Carb per Serving	GL per Serving
Eggs, large	[0]	2	0	0
Enercal Plus™ (Wyeth-Ayerst)	61	8 oz	40	24
English Muffin™ bread (Natural Ovens)	77	1 oz	14	11
Ensure™, vanilla drink	48	8 oz	34	16
Ensure™ bar, chocolate fudge brownie	43	1.4 oz	20	8
Ensure Plus™, vanilla drink	40	8 oz	47	19
Ensure Pudding™, old-fashioned vanilla	36	4 oz	26	9

F

FOOD	GI Value	Nominal Serving Size	Net Carb per Serving	GL per Serving
Fanta®, orange soft drink	68	8 oz	34	23
Fettuccine, egg, cooked	32	1½ cups	46	15
Figs, dried	61	3	26	16
Fish	[0]	4 oz	0	0
Fish sticks	38	3.5 oz	19	7
Flan/crème caramel	65	½ cup	73	47
French baguette, white, plain	95	1 oz	15	15

[0] indicates that the food has so little carbohydrate that the GI value cannot be tested. The GL, therefore, is 0.

FOOD	GI Value	Nominal Serving Size	Net Carb per Serving	GL per Serving
French fries, frozen, reheated in microwave	75	30 pcs	29	22
French green beans, cooked	[0]	½ cup	0	0
French vanilla cake made from mix, with vanilla frosting	42	4 oz	58	24
French vanilla ice cream, premium, 16% fat	38	½ cup	14	5
Froot Loops™, breakfast cereal	69	1 cup	26	18
Frosted Flakes™, breakfast cereal	55	1 cup	26	15
Fructose, pure	19	1 Tbsp	10	2
Fruit cocktail, canned, light syrup	55	½ cup	16	9
Fruit leather	61	2 pcs	24	15

G

FOOD	GI Value	Nominal Serving Size	Net Carb per Serving	GL per Serving
Gatorade™ (orange) sports drink	89	8 oz	15	13
Gin	[0]	1 oz	0	0
Glucerna™, vanilla (Abbott)	31	8 oz	23	7
Glucose (dextrose)	99	1 Tbsp	10	10
Glucose tablets	102	3 pcs	15	15
Gluten-free corn pasta	78	1½ cups	42	32
Gluten-free multigrain bread	79	1 oz	13	10
Gluten-free rice and corn pasta	76	1½ cups	49	37
Gluten-free spaghetti, rice and split pea, canned in tomato sauce	68	8 oz	27	19
Gluten-free split pea and soy pasta shells	29	1½ cups	31	9
Gluten-free white bread, sliced	80	1 oz	15	12
Glutinous (sticky) rice, white, cooked	92	⅔ cup	48	44
Gnocchi	68	6 oz	48	33
Grapefruit, fresh, medium	25	1 half	11	3
Grapefruit juice, unsweetened	48	8 oz	20	9
Grape-Nuts® (Post), breakfast cereal	75	¼ cup	21	16

[0] indicates that the food has so little carbohydrate that the GI value cannot be tested. The GL, therefore, is 0.

FOOD	GI Value	Nominal Serving Size	Net Carb per Serving	GL per Serving
Grapes, black, fresh	59	¾ cup	18	11
Grapes, green, fresh	46	¾ cup	18	8
Green peas	48	⅓ cup	7	3
Green pea soup, canned	66	8 oz	41	27

H

FOOD	GI Value	Nominal Serving Size	Net Carb per Serving	GL per Serving
Hamburger bun	61	1.5 oz	22	13
Happiness™ (cinnamon, raisin, pecan bread) (Natural Ovens)	63	1 oz	14	9
Hazelnuts	[0]	1.75 oz	0	0
Healthy Choice™ Hearty 100% Whole Grain	62	1 oz	14	9
Healthy Choice™ Hearty 7-Grain	55	1 oz	14	8
Honey	55	1 Tbsp	18	10
Hot cereal, apple & cinnamon, dry (Con Agra)	37	1.2 oz	22	8
Hot cereal, unflavored, dry (Con Agra)	25	1.2 oz	19	5
Hunger Filler™, whole-grain bread (Natural Ovens)	59	1 oz	13	7

I

FOOD	GI Value	Nominal Serving Size	Net Carb per Serving	GL per Serving
Ice cream, low-fat, vanilla, "light"	50	½ cup	9	5
Ice cream, premium, French vanilla, 16% fat	38	½ cup	14	5
Ice cream, premium, "ultra chocolate," 15% fat	37	½ cup	14	5
Ice cream, regular fat	61	½ cup	20	12
Instant potato, mashed	97	¾ cup	20	17
Instant rice, white, cooked 6 min	87	¾ cup	42	36
Ironman PR® bar, chocolate	39	2.3 oz	26	10

[0] indicates that the food has so little carbohydrate that the GI value cannot be tested. The GL, therefore, is 0.

FOOD	GI Value	Nominal Serving Size	Net Carb per Serving	GL per Serving
J				
Jam, apricot fruit spread, reduced sugar	55	1½ Tbsps	13	7
Jam, strawberry	51	1½ Tbsps	20	10
Jasmine rice, white, cooked	109	1 cup	42	46
Jelly beans	78	10 large	28	22
K				
Kaiser roll	73	1 half	16	12
Kavli™ Norwegian crispbread	71	5 pcs	16	12
Kidney beans, canned	52	⅔ cup	17	9
Kidney beans, cooked	23	⅔ cup	25	6
Kiwi fruit	58	4 oz	12	7
Kudos® Whole Grain Bars, chocolate chip	62	1.8 oz	32	20
L				
Lactose, pure	46	1 Tbsp	10	5
Lamb	[0]	4 oz	0	0
Leafy vegetables (spinach, arugula, etc.), raw	[0]	1½ cups	0	0
L.E.A.N Fibergy™ bar, Harvest Oat	45	1.75 oz	29	13
L.E.A.N Life long Nutribar™, Chocolate Crunch	32	1.5 oz	19	6
L.E.A.N Life long Nutribar™, Peanut Crunch	30	1.5 oz	19	6
L.E.A.N Nutrimeal™, drink powder, Dutch Chocolate	26	8 oz	13	3
Lemonade, reconstituted	66	8 oz	20	13
Lentil soup, canned	44	9 oz	21	9
Lentils, brown, cooked	29	¾ cup	18	5
Lentils, green, cooked	30	¾ cup	17	5
Lentils, red, cooked	26	¾ cup	18	5

[0] indicates that the food has so little carbohydrate that the GI value cannot be tested. The GL, therefore, is 0.

FOOD	GI Value	Nominal Serving Size	Net Carb per Serving	GL per Serving
Lettuce	[0]	4 leaves	0	0
Life Savers®, peppermint candy	70	18 pcs	30	21
Light rye bread	68	1 oz	14	10
Lima beans, baby, frozen	32	¾ cup	30	10
Linguine pasta, thick, cooked	46	1½ cups	48	22
Linguine pasta, thin, cooked	52	1½ cups	45	23
Long-grain rice, cooked 10 min	61	1 cup	36	22
Lychees, canned in syrup, drained	79	4 oz	20	16

M

FOOD	GI Value	Nominal Serving Size	Net Carb per Serving	GL per Serving
M & M's®, peanut	33	15 pcs	17	6
Macadamia nuts	[0]	1.75 oz	0	0
Macaroni and cheese, made from mix	64	1 cup	51	32
Macaroni, cooked	47	1¼ cups	48	23
Maltose	105	1 Tbsp	10	11
Mango	51	4 oz	15	8
Maple syrup, pure Canadian	54	1 Tbsp	18	10
Marmalade, orange	48	1½ Tbsps	20	9
Mars Bar®	68	2 oz	40	27
Melba toast, Old London	70	6 pcs	23	16
METRx® bar (vanilla)	74	3.6 oz	50	37
Milk Arrowroot™ cookies	69	5	18	12
Millet, cooked	71	⅔ cup	36	25
Mini Wheats™, whole-wheat breakfast cereal	58	12 pcs	21	12
Mousse, butterscotch, 1.9% fat	36	1.75 oz	10	4
Mousse, chocolate, 2% fat	31	1.75 oz	11	3
Mousse, hazelnut, 2.4% fat	36	1.75 oz	10	4
Mousse, mango, 1.8% fat	33	1.75 oz	11	4
Mousse, mixed berry, 2.2% fat	36	1.75 oz	10	4
Mousse, strawberry, 2.3% fat	32	1.75 oz	10	3

[0] indicates that the food has so little carbohydrate that the GI value cannot be tested. The GL, therefore, is 0.

FOOD	GI Value	Nominal Serving Size	Net Carb per Serving	GL per Serving
Muesli bar containing dried fruit	61	1 oz	21	13
Muesli bread, made from mix in bread oven (Con Agra)	54	1 oz	12	7
Muesli, gluten-free, with low-fat milk	39	1 oz	19	7
Muesli, Swiss Formula	56	1 oz	16	9
Muesli, toasted	43	1 oz	17	7
Multi-Grain 9-Grain bread	43	1 oz	14	6

N

FOOD	GI Value	Nominal Serving Size	Net Carb per Serving	GL per Serving
Navy beans, canned	38	5 oz	31	12
Nesquik™, chocolate dissolved in low-fat milk, no-sugar-added	41	8 oz	11	5
Nesquik™, strawberry dissolved in low-fat milk, no-sugar-added	35	8 oz	12	4
New creamer potato, canned	65	5 oz	18	12
New creamer potato, unpeeled and cooked 20 min	78	5 oz	21	16
Noodles, instant "two-minute" (Maggi®)	46	1½ cups	40	19
Noodles, mung bean (Lungkow beanthread), dried, cooked	39	1½ cups	45	18
Noodles, rice, fresh, cooked	40	1½ cups	39	15
Nutella®, chocolate hazelnut spread	33	1 Tbsp	12	4
Nutrigrain™, breakfast cereal	66	1 cup	15	10
Nutty Natural™, whole-grain bread (Natural Ovens)	59	1 oz	12	7

O

FOOD	GI Value	Nominal Serving Size	Net Carb per Serving	GL per Serving
Oat bran, raw	55	2 Tbsp	5	3
Oatmeal, cooked 1 min	66	1 cup	26	17
Oatmeal cookies	55	4 small	21	12
Orange juice, unsweetened, reconstituted	53	8 oz	18	9

[0] indicates that the food has so little carbohydrate that the GI value cannot be tested. The GL, therefore, is 0.

FOOD	GI Value	Nominal Serving Size	Net Carb per Serving	GL per Serving
Orange, fresh, medium	42	4 oz	11	5

P

FOOD	GI Value	Nominal Serving Size	Net Carb per Serving	GL per Serving
Pancakes, buckwheat, gluten-free, made from mix	102	2 4" pancakes	22	22
Pancakes, made from mix	67	2 4" pancakes	58	39
Papaya, fresh	59	4 oz	8	5
Parsnips	97	½ cup	12	12
Pastry	59	2 oz	26	15
Pea soup, canned	66	8 oz	41	27
Peach, canned in heavy syrup	58	½ cup	26	15
Peach, canned in light syrup	52	½ cup	18	9
Peach, fresh, large	42	4 oz	11	5
Peanuts	14	1.75 oz	6	1
Pear halves, canned in natural juice	43	½ cup	13	5
Pear, fresh	38	4 oz	11	4
Peas, green, frozen, cooked	48	½ cup	7	3
Pecans	[0]	1.75 oz	0	0
Pepper, fresh, green or red	[0]	3 oz	0	0
Pineapple, fresh	66	4 oz	10	6
Pineapple juice, unsweetened	46	8 oz	34	15
Pinto beans, canned	45	⅔ cup	22	10
Pinto beans, dried, cooked	39	¾ cup	26	10
Pita bread, white	57	1 oz	17	10
Pizza, cheese	60	1 slice	27	16
Pizza, Super Supreme, pan (11.4% fat)	36	1 slice	24	9
Pizza, Super Supreme, thin and crispy (13.2% fat)	30	1 slice	22	7
Plums, fresh	39	2 medium	12	5
Pop Tarts™, double chocolate	70	1.8 oz pastry	36	25
Popcorn, plain, cooked in microwave oven	72	1½ cups	11	8

[0] indicates that the food has so little carbohydrate that the GI value cannot be tested. The GL, therefore, is 0.

FOOD	GI Value	Nominal Serving Size	Net Carb per Serving	GL per Serving
Pork	[0]	4 oz	0	0
Potato chips, plain, salted	54	2 oz	21	11
Potato, baked	85	5 oz	30	26
Potato, microwaved	82	5 oz	33	27
Pound cake (Sara Lee)	54	2 oz	28	15
PowerBar® (chocolate)	57	2.3 oz	42	24
Premium soda crackers	74	5 crackers	17	12
Pretzels	83	1 oz	20	16
Prunes, pitted	29	6	33	10
Pudding, instant, chocolate, made with whole milk	47	½ cup	24	11
Pudding, instant, vanilla, made with whole milk	40	½ cup	24	10
Puffed crispbread	81	1 oz	19	15
Puffed rice cakes, white	82	3 cakes	21	17
Puffed Wheat, breakfast cereal	80	2 cups	21	17
Pumpernickel rye kernel bread	41	1 oz	12	5
Pumpkin	75	3 oz	4	3
R				
Raisin Bran™, breakfast cereal	61	½ cup	19	12
Raisins	64	½ cup	44	28
Ravioli, meat-filled, cooked	39	6.5 oz	38	15
Red wine	[0]	3.5 oz	0	0
Red-skinned potato, peeled and microwaved on high for 6–7.5 min	79	5 oz	18	14
Red-skinned potato, peeled, boiled 35 min	88	5 oz	18	16
Red-skinned potato, peeled, mashed	91	5 oz	20	18
Resource Diabetic™, nutritional support product, vanilla (Novartis)	34	8 oz	23	8
Rice and corn pasta, gluten-free	76	1½ cups	49	37

[0] indicates that the food has so little carbohydrate that the GI value cannot be tested. The GL, therefore, is 0.

FOOD	GI Value	Nominal Serving Size	Net Carb per Serving	GL per Serving
Rice bran, extruded	19	1 oz	14	3
Rice cakes, white	82	3 cakes	21	17
Rice Krispies™, breakfast cereal	82	1¼ cups	26	22
Rice Krispies Treat™ bar	63	1 oz	24	15
Rice noodles, fresh, cooked	40	1½ cups	39	15
Rice, parboiled	72	1 cup	36	26
Rice pasta, brown, cooked 16 min	92	1½ cups	38	35
Rice vermicelli	58	1½ cups	39	22
Rolled oats	42	1 cup	21	9
Roll-Ups®, processed fruit snack	99	1 oz	25	24
Roman (cranberry) beans, fresh, cooked	46	¾ cup	18	8
Russet, baked potato	85	5 oz	30	26
Rutabaga, fresh, cooked	72	5 oz	10	7
Rye bread	58	1 oz	14	8
Ryvita® crackers	69	3 crackers	16	11
S				
Salami	[0]	4 oz	0	0
Salmon	[0]	4 oz	0	0
Sausages, fried	28	3.5 oz	3	1
Scones, plain	92	1 oz	9	8
Sebago potato, peeled, cooked	87	5 oz	17	14
Seeded rye bread	55	1 oz	13	7
Semolina, cooked (dry)	55	⅓ cup	50	28
Shellfish (shrimp, crab, lobster, etc.)	[0]	4 oz	0	0
Sherry	[0]	2 oz	0	0
Shortbread cookies	64	1 oz	16	10
Shredded Wheat™, breakfast cereal	75	⅔ cup	20	15
Shredded Wheat™ biscuits	62	1 oz	18	11
Skim milk	32	8 oz	13	4

[0] indicates that the food has so little carbohydrate that the GI value cannot be tested. The GL, therefore, is 0.

FOOD	GI Value	Nominal Serving Size	Net Carb per Serving	GL per Serving
Skittles®	70	45 pcs	45	32
Smacks™, breakfast cereal	71	¾ cup	23	11
Smoothie, raspberry (Con Agra)	33	8 oz	41	14
Snack bar, Apple Cinnamon (Con Agra)	40	1.75 oz	29	12
Snack bar, Peanut Butter & Choc-Chip (Con Agra)	37	1.75 oz	27	10
Snickers® bar	68	2.2 oz	35	23
Soda Crackers, Premium	74	5 crackers	17	12
Soft drink, Coca Cola®	53	8 oz	26	14
Soft drink, Fanta®, orange	68	8 oz	34	23
Sourdough rye	48	1 oz	12	6
Sourdough wheat	54	1 oz	14	8
Soy & Flaxseed bread (mix in bread oven) (Con Agra)	50	1 oz	10	5
Soybeans, canned	14	1 cup	6	1
Soybeans, dried, cooked	20	1 cup	6	1
Spaghetti, durum wheat, cooked 20 min	64	1½ cups	43	27
Spaghetti, gluten-free, rice and split pea, canned in tomato sauce	68	8 oz	27	19
Spaghetti, white, cooked 5 min	38	1½ cups	48	18
Spaghetti, whole wheat, cooked 5 min	32	1½ cups	44	14
Special K™, breakfast cereal	69	1 cup	21	14
Spirali pasta, durum wheat, al dente	43	1½ cups	44	19
Split pea and soy pasta shells, gluten-free	29	1½ cups	31	9
Split-pea soup	60	1 cup	27	16
Split peas, yellow, cooked 20 min	32	¾ cup	19	6
Sponge cake, plain	46	2 oz	36	17
Squash, raw	[0]	⅔ cup	0	0
Star pastina, white, cooked 5 min	38	1½ cups	48	18

[0] indicates that the food has so little carbohydrate that the GI value cannot be tested. The GL, therefore, is 0.

FOOD	GI Value	Nominal Serving Size	Net Carb per Serving	GL per Serving
Stay Trim™, whole-grain bread (Natural Ovens)	70	1 oz	15	10
Stoned Wheat Thins	67	14 crackers	17	12
Strawberries, fresh	40	4 oz	3	1
Strawberry jam	51	1½ Tbsps	20	10
Strawberry shortcake	42	2.2 oz	40	17
Stuffing, bread	74	1 oz	21	16
Sucrose	68	1 Tbsp	10	7
Super Supreme pizza, pan (11.4% fat)	36	1 slice	24	9
Super Supreme pizza, thin and crispy (13.2% fat)	30	1 slice	22	7
Sushi, salmon	48	3.5 oz	36	17
Sweet corn, whole kernel, canned, diet-pack, drained	46	1 cup	28	13
Sweet potato, cooked	44	5 oz	25	11
T				
Taco shells, baked	68	2 shells	12	8
Tapioca, cooked with milk	81	¾ cup	18	14
Tofu-based frozen dessert, chocolate with high-fructose (24%) corn syrup	115	1.75 oz	9	10
Tomato juice, canned, no added sugar	38	8 oz	9	4
Tomato soup	38	1 cup	17	6
Tortollini, cheese	50	6.5 oz	21	10
Tortilla chips, plain, salted	63	1.75 oz	26	17
Total™, breakfast cereal	76	¾ cup	22	17
Tuna	[0]	4 oz	0	0
Twix® Cookie Bar, caramel	44	2 cookies	39	17
U				
Ultra chocolate ice cream, premium, 15% fat	37	½ cup	14	5

[0] indicates that the food has so little carbohydrate that the GI value cannot be tested. The GL, therefore, is 0.

FOOD	GI Value	Nominal Serving Size	Net Carb per Serving	GL per Serving
Ultracal™ with fiber (Mead Johnson)	40	8 oz	29	12
V				
Vanilla cake made from mix, with vanilla frosting	42	4 oz	58	24
Vanilla pudding, instant, made with whole milk	40	½ cup	24	10
Vanilla wafers	77	6 cookies	18	14
Veal	[0]	4 oz	0	0
Vermicelli, white, cooked	35	1½ cups	44	16
W				
Waffles, Aunt Jemima®	76	1 4" waffle	13	10
Walnuts	[0]	1.75 oz	0	0
Water crackers	78	7 crackers	18	14
Watermelon, fresh	72	4 oz	6	4
Weet-Bix™, breakfast cereal	69	2 biscuits	17	12
Wheaties™, breakfast cereal	82	1 cup	21	17
Whiskey	[0]	1 oz	0	0
White bread	70	1 oz	14	10
White rice, instant, cooked 6 min	87	1 cup	42	36
White wine	[0]	3.5 oz	0	0
100% Whole Grain™ bread (Natural Ovens)	51	1 oz	13	7
Whole milk	31	8 oz	12	4
Whole-wheat bread	77	1 oz	12	9
Wonder™ white bread	80	1 oz	14	11
X				
Xylitol	8	1 Tbsp	10	1
Y				
Yam, peeled, cooked	37	5 oz	36	13

[0] indicates that the food has so little carbohydrate that the GI value cannot be tested. The GL, therefore, is 0.

FOOD	GI Value	Nominal Serving Size	Net Carb per Serving	GL per Serving
Yogurt, low-fat, wild strawberry	31	8 oz	34	11
Yogurt, low-fat, with fruit and artificial sweetener	14	8 oz	15	2
Yogurt, low-fat, with fruit and sugar	33	8 oz	35	12

[0] indicates that the food has so little carbohydrate that the GI value cannot be tested. The GL, therefore, is 0.

FOR MORE INFORMATION

To find a dietitian:
The American Dietetic Association
120 S. Riverside Plaza
Suite 2000
Chicago, IL 60606
Phone: 1-800-877-1600
www.eatright.org

**To order Natural Ovens bread
(available through mail-order only):**
Natural Ovens Bakery
PO Box 730
Manitowoc, WI 54221-0730
Phone: 1-800-772-0730
www.naturalovens.com

To order Fifty50 Foods:

Fifty50 Foods, Inc.
c/o Spectrum Foods, Inc.
PO Box 3493
Springfield, IL 62708
Phone: 1-800-238-8090
www.specialtyfoodpantries.com
www.fifty50.com

GLYCEMIC INDEX TESTING

*I*F YOU ARE a food manufacturer, you may be interested in having the glycemic index value of some of your products tested on a fee-for-service basis. For more information, contact:

Sydney University Glycemic Index Research Service (SUGiRS)
Department of Biochemistry
University of Sydney
NSW 2006 Australia
Fax: (61) (2) 9351-6022
E-mail: j.brandmiller@staff.usyd.edu.au

ACKNOWLEDGMENTS

WE WOULD LIKE to thank Linda Rao, M.Ed., for her editorial work on the American edition.

ABOUT THE AUTHORS

JENNIE BRAND-MILLER, PH.D., is Professor of Human Nutrition in the Human Nutrition Unit, School of Molecular and Microbial Biosciences at the University of Sydney, and President of the Nutrition Society of Australia. She has taught postgraduate students of nutrition and dietetics at the University of Sydney for over twenty-four years and currently leads a team of twelve research scientists, whose interests focus on all aspects of carbohydrate—diet and diabetes, the glycemic index of foods, insulin resistance, lactose intolerance, and oligosaccharides in infant nutrition. She has published sixteen books and 140 journal articles and is the co-author of all books in the Glucose Revolution series.

■

JOHANNA BURANI, M.S., R.D., C.D.E., is a Registered Dietitian and Certified Diabetes Educator with more than thirteen years' experience in nutritional counseling. The co-author of *The Glucose Revolution Life Plan* and author of *Good Carbs, Bad Carbs*, as well as several other books and professional manuals, she specializes in designing individual meal plans based on low-GI food choices. She lives in Mendham, New Jersey.

■

KAYE FOSTER-POWELL, M. NUTR. & DIET., is an accredited practicing dietitian with extensive experience in diabetes management. She has conducted research into the glycemic index of foods and its practical applications over the last fifteen years. Currently she is a dietitian with Wentworth Area Diabetes Services in New South Wales and consults on all aspects of the glycemic index. She is the co-author of all books in the Glucose Revolution series.

■

LINDA RAO, M.ED., a freelance writer and editor, has been writing and researching health topics for the past thirteen years. Her work has appeared in several national publications, including *Prevention*, *Organic Style*, and *Better Homes & Gardens*. She serves as a contributing editor for *Prevention* magazine and is the co-adapter, with Johanna Burani, of all the titles in The Glucose Revolution Pocket Guide Series. She lives in Allentown, Pennsylvania.

Also Available

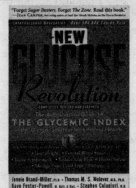

"Forget *Sugar Busters*. Forget *The Zone*. Read this book."
—JEAN CARPER, *best-selling author of* Food: Your Miracle Medicine *and* Your Miracle Brain

ISBN 1-56924-506-1 • $15.95

New York Times bestseller

THE NEW GLUCOSE REVOLUTION

The Authoritative Guide to the Glycemic Index—the Dietary Solution for Lifelong Health

Written by the world's leading authorities on the subject, whose findings are supported by hundreds of studies from Harvard University's School of Public Health and other leading research centers, *The New Glucose Revolution* shows how and why eating low-GI foods has major health benefits for everybody seeking to establish a way of eating for lifelong health.

THE GLUCOSE REVOLUTION LIFE PLAN

Discover how to make the glycemic index —the most significant dietary finding of the last 25 years— the foundation for a lifetime of healthy eating

More than 60,000 copies sold!

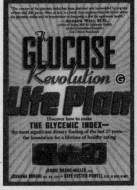

ISBN 1-56924-609-2 • $18.95

Both an introduction to the benefits of low-GI foods and an essential source for those already familiar with the concept, *The Glucose Revolution Life Plan* presents the glycemic index within the context of today's full nutrition picture.

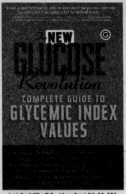

THE NEW GLUCOSE REVOLUTION COMPLETE GUIDE TO GLYCEMIC INDEX VALUES

The *Only* Authoritative, Comprehensive, Up-to-Date Guide to Glycemic Index Values—A Companion to *The New Glucose Revolution*

With GI values for hundreds of foods and beverages, *The New GLucose Revolution Complete Guide to Glycemic Index Values* makes it easier than ever to ascertain a food's GI value. Each of the three easy-to-read tables in this book lists a food's GI value, serving size, net carbohydrate per serving, and glycemic load, which is clearly explained.

WHAT MAKES MY BLOOD GLUCOSE GO UP . . . AND DOWN?

And 101 Other Frequently Asked Questions About Your Blood Glucose Levels

In this accessible, informative book, *The New Glucose Revolution*'s Jennie Brand-Miller and Kaye Foster-Powell team up with leading diabetes journalist Rick Mendosa to answer the most frequently asked questions about your blood glucose levels, from "What is a normal blood glucose level?" to "What should I eat when I crave something sweet?"

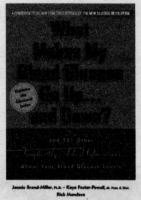

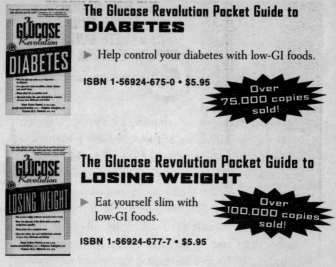
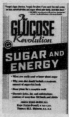
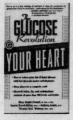

Food manufacturers are showing increasing interest in having the GI values of their products measured. Some are already including the GI value of foods on food labels. As more and more research highlights the benefits of low-GI foods, consumers and dietitians are writing and telephoning food companies and diabetes organizations asking for GI data. This symbol has been registered in several countries, including the United States and Australia, to indicate that a food has been properly GI tested—in real people, not in a test tube—and also makes a positive contribution to nutrition. You can find out more about the program at www.gisymbol.com.au.

As consumers, you have a right to information about the nutrients and physiological effects of foods. You have a right to know the GI value of a food and to know it has been tested using appropriate standardized methodology.